Boomer Smarts
Boomer Power

To Deb,
A Boomer who definitely has the Boomer Smarts! You raise the Bar. Deb, + I am so fortunate that I know you.
XXOXO
Mitzi
3-2014

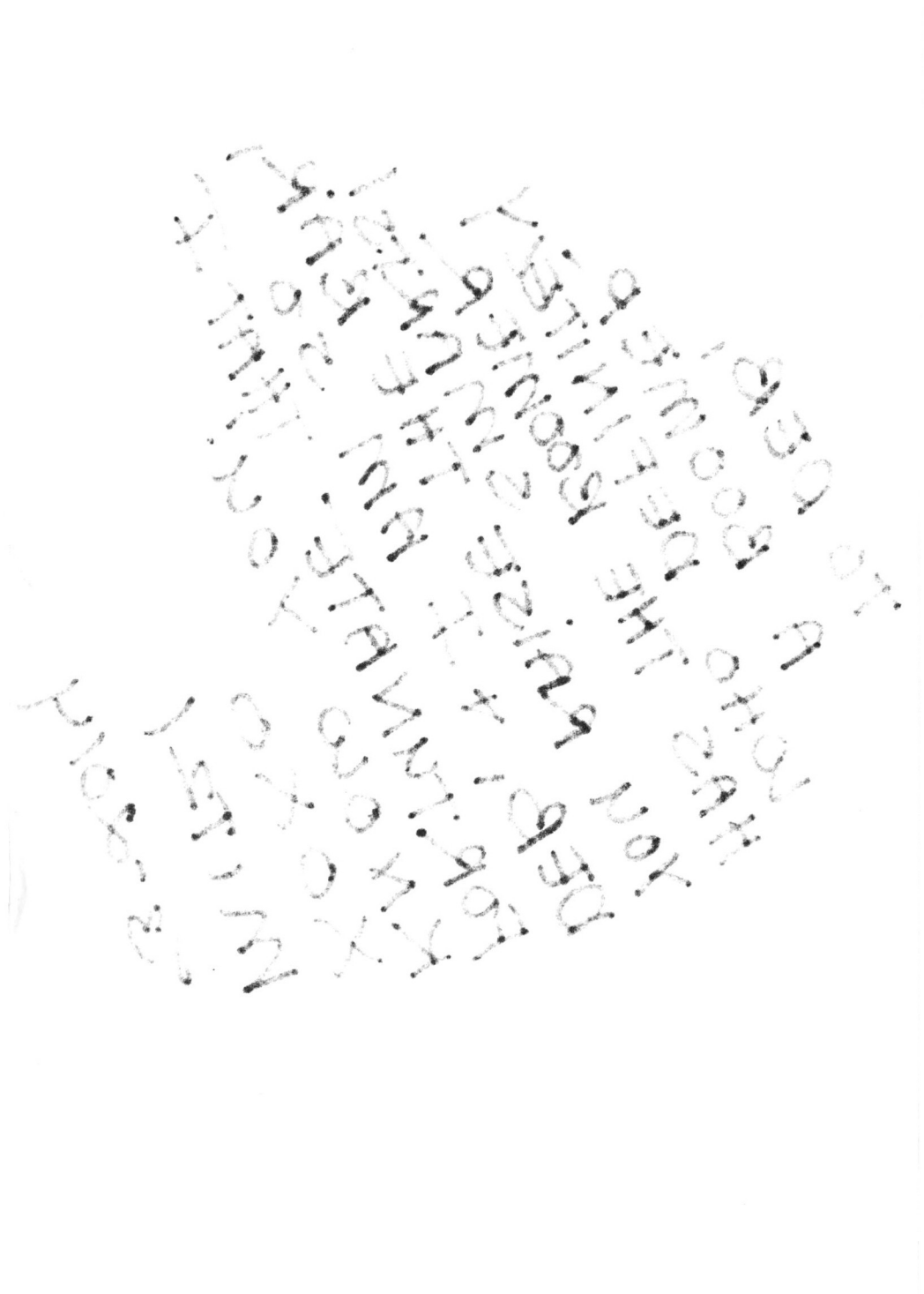

TO DEB, BOOMER &
YOUR BOOK IS DEFINITELY
THE BOOK DEFINITELY A
HIT BUT I WANT
YOU TO KNOW IT
DEB PRINTS KNOW
COME VISIT
MISSY

Boomer Smarts
Boomer Power

Six Steps to Living Your Best for the Rest of Your Life

Mitzi Beach

www.MitziBeach.com

This book and the information contained herein are for informative purposes only. The information in this book is distributed on an "As Is" basis, without warranty. The author makes no legal claims, express or implied, and the material is not meant to substitute for legal, medical, or financial counsel.

Nothing contained in this book is intended to be, or should be considered as, medical advice or a substitute for medical advice, diagnosis, or treatment. You should not disregard any advice provided to you by your medical or mental health providers, or delay seeking treatment from them, based on any information contained in this book.

The author, publisher, and/or copyright holder assume no responsibility for the loss or damage caused, or allegedly caused, directly or indirectly, by the use of information contained in this book. The author and publisher specifically dis-claim any liability incurred from the use or application of the contents of this book.

All rights reserved. No part of this book may be reproduced or transmitted in any form or by any means, electronic, mechanical, photocopying, recording, or otherwise, without the prior written permission of the publisher.

Throughout this book trademarked names are referenced. Rather than putting a trademark symbol by every occurrence of a trademarked name, we state that we are using the names in an editorial fashion only and to the benefit of the trademark owner with no intention of infringement of the trademark.

Copyright © 2013 Mitzi Beach
All Rights Reserved

Printed in the United States of America

ISBN-13: 978-1493715527
ISBN-10: 1493715526

*I dedicate this book to my number one
and to my favorite Boomer, my husband Bob;
and to my parents, Ellen and Jim Garrett.
To these three, I owe it all*

Six *Boomer Smarts* Steps to Living Your Best

Spaces. *In our living spaces.*

Mindsets. *In our mindsets on aging.*

Attitudes. *In our attitudes on aging.*

Routines. *In our routine lifestyles.*

Togetherness. *In our community.*

Spirituality. *In our spiritual lives.*

Contents

Acknowledgements 11

Foreword 13

Chapter 1. Spaces 17

   Why We Did the Outrageous
   in Our Late Boomer Years 17

   Cypress: Our Boomer Smart Home 22

   What the Boomer Really Wants in a Home,
   But Who Is Listening? 34

   Bonus List for the Really Smart Boomer 40

   Boomer Smart Stories 42
      Cindy Carnahan
      Kelly Kole
      Geri Higgins

Chapter 2. Mindsets 61

   Make Up Thy Boomer Mind
   to Be Boomer Smart 61

   Live Your Boomer Wisdom
   By Knowing and Doing Boomer Smarts 67

Me, Refused? You Have to Be Kidding! 70

Where the Boomer Mind Goes
the Boomer Will Surely Follow 72

Knowing Without Doing Is Not
Living a Boomer Smart Life 73

Questions for Chapter 2: Mindsets 76

Boomer Smart Stories 77
Leslie Carothers
Lynne Barton Bier

Chapter 3. Attitudes 93

Ageless Aging with a
Boomer Smart Attitude 93

Garbage In, Garbage Out 98

Boomers Get to Choose 102

Boomer Smart Stories 106
Cynthia Bogart
Barbara Barton

Chapter 4. Routines 141

Boomer Smarts: Healthy Aging Is
75% Lifestyle, 25% Genetics 141

Healthy Cooking and Eating Routines 147

Boomer Smart Balance and Wholeness 156

Boomer Smart Wellness Meter 164

Boomer Smart Stories 168
Mary Baldwin

Chapter 5. Togetherness 183

Boomers with Boomer Smarts
Live to Give 183

Leaving a Legacy of Influence 185

Boomer Smart Stories 189
Doreen Hanna

Chapter 6. Spirituality 203

Connecting the Dots: How Boomer Smarts
Enable Boomers to Live
in Boomer Power 203

Where We Are Now 212

Boomer Power 215

Boomer Smart Stories 216
Leslie Wood
Karen Porter

Epilogue: What's Next? 233

About the Author 235

Acknowledgments

I imagine that only authors using ghost writers do not need or have layers of remarkable people behind them pushing, challenging, and encouraging them to keep on keeping on. Here are my remarkable people that I so want to acknowledge for their part in actually making me an author!

Joan Hearn and Dee Schmidt have poured into my life and career as my mentors and my lifecoaches for years and years, expecting nothing in return but to see me go higher and higher.

Diana Peden, Linda McMillan, Joey Pohl, Leslie Carothers, Joanna Myhre, Debbie Delaney, Laura Hannon, Debbie Lundrum, and Catherine Mutheey were the loyal and prayerful friends that never doubted my calling to bring my passion for the Boomers to life in print.

The remarkable women that agreed without hesitation to do the book interviews in such sincere authenticity and vulnerability that will enrich us all with their life stories.

And what could be more special in your later years than to have your siblings behind you, and I certainly did with my sister, Kim Barnes, and my brother, Jim Garrett.

And to the strategy genius of Monaica Ledell and Bob Regnerus, and the technical genius of Andrew Ledell; most would otherwise never ever know of Mitzi Beach or this book.

And to the fine work of editing by Joanne Asala, who

even researched fonts for us Boomers.

To Gavin Peters, the photographer for my own website, www.MitziBeach.com, book cover, and parts of our home; he is the genius behind these photos. Ryan Hendrix took the early photos of our home Cypress, showing his creative talents through his camera lenses.

And, of course, to my amazing family of six adult "children and spouses" and nine grandchildren who, after my faith, are the apple of my eye.

And then there is my husband, Bob. Only he truly knows all the years we sacrificed together to not only restore our home Cypress, but to truly believe we are on a path of destiny…yet unknown and yet certain.

To all of these remarkable people, I thank them beyond what words can express.

— *Mitzi Beach*

Foreword

I was an eighteen-year-old freshman at my orientation at Ohio University. My hometown of Salem, Ohio, had 12,000 people, and Ohio U had a daunting enrollment of 18,000 students. I had never been on an airplane, never been away from home other than with family or close classmates to go camping. Heck, I'd never even had a babysitter because we did everything with family...even vacations.

I wasn't too intimated by being away from home with all these strangers until, sitting with all my other freshmen classmates during orientation, some dean said, "Look to the person on your left, look to the person on your right. One of you will not be here to start your second semester."

What?? Why would he say that to me? I am a nice person and I am already homesick and scared of all that I don't know about being so far from home, and now they want to get rid of me...why?

It was simply because there were too many of us. Ohio University, like other state schools, had at that time a policy to admit all state students who applied, knowing many would not make it through till second semester. I didn't know it was just simply policy to deal with sheer numbers, I was freaked out!

And "the beat goes on," as Sonny and Cher sang in the most popular song known during many Boomers' lives... "The beat goes on" with America not being prepared for the vast numbers of us Boomers...even now as we enter into Medicare, Social Security, retirement, new and different housing needs and wants, and yet...

It is like no one knew we existed or had not prepared for our huge numbers, right?

I wrote this book because America is not ready for us in our next stage of life. Perhaps even sadder is that Boomers, without the vision of believing we are not like former generations, are not ready either for our next stage of life.

But being optimistic, and like a true Baby Boomer, I think, "Well, we have changed every single decade of our Boomer history, why not change the way we deal with getting older?"

Without a doubt, I believe that aging better for Boomers involves being prepared in our homes, our health, and in our attitudes. We need to be proactive in demanding that our futures look different and not simply reactive, expecting the same pattern of aging as what other generations have experienced. Oh no, this old stinking thinking on aging is not for us believing Boomers! No, not for us Boomers who believe we will age like no other generation before us. Watch and see this huge movement unfolding in America to change the face of aging—and I'm not talking plastic surgery—by believing Boomers being a model for those who are grasping never-before-seen living spaces, healthy lifestyles, and "life-is-good" attitudes.

Just take how we visualize our homes for Boomers in their futures. I am a huge proponent that our homes propel us to a greater level of potential if we create sanctuary spaces that allow us to not just exist, but to live life to its fullest potential.

Gail Doby, cofounder and chief visionary for Design Success University, states: "Your house is not a home until it expresses your soul."

Foreword

Exactly! Life at this stage should be celebrated and expressed through our homes and in our healthy lifestyles and in our sassy, watch-me-now attitudes.

I wrote this book for the Boomer Believers and not for the Boomers determined to stay stuck in old paradigms in their minds, homes, and their health.

This is for those mover and shaker Boomers who visualize their futures as the most freeing and exciting times of their unique Boomer lives. And yet, major questions hang precariously in their Boomer minds. What will my health look like? What will my living spaces be like?

Well, now is the time for these Boomers to celebrate not only where they are presently but also where they are going. And it can be good, really, really good. But…

To step up and live the best years of a Boomer life, the answer lies in knowing and doing Boomer Smarts.

To Boomers everywhere:

"Live your Wisdom" by and through being a Boomer Smart Boomer. Become part of this exciting movement that is going to forever change aging in America.

And this is exactly why I felt compelled to write this book: To position Boomers to live the best rest of their lives, moving gracefully, and yes, even joyfully into this awesome stage of Boomerhood, whether that means in our fifties or in our sixties and beyond.

We are the Baby Boomers and we will indeed change the way America ages…you'll see.

Chapter 1
Spaces

Why We Did the Outrageous in Our Late Boomer Years

My "empty-nest/launching adult kids" stage was so much more than our kids growing up and leaving. I painfully knew that our lives were being forever changed. Not only was our nest empty, but my heart was empty, too.

Nothing was working in my life at this empty-nest stage the way I thought that it would after all those HARD years of raising kids, keeping my interior design business "fed" with tons of my energy, staying in the fifty percent of those not divorced, trying to make things work better...always trying...always trying.

And one day I simply and profoundly thought, "This life and this identity sucks!"

Oh, most definitely did we have all those memories of raising our twin sons and one daughter through fun, adventurous, bonding years that will forever be imprinted on my heart and mind. Those awesome, wonderful, heartfelt years of all the stages of raising a family, cherished beyond what I could ever have imagined in joy and love truly experienced.

But when the house emptied out, and the "launching stage," as I call it, began, it all changed on a dime (as

I say when things happen suddenly), and I was totally unprepared for how to handle it. I had no idea what to do with all these feelings, especially when some of my friends were just elated at being empty nesters. They certainly could not relate to my utter hopelessness at the "now what?" question.

That "now what?" question can be haunting for us Boomers. This is how I answered that "now what?" question, and why my husband and I did what we did in our late Boomer years.

Now, being a true rebellious Baby Boomer, staying in this quicksand of self-pity eventually and laboriously turned to righteous anger that got my fire back and my Boomer "don't tell me this is all there is to my life" self-talk. No way was I going to stay here in this pit of despair and experience such unidentified frustration all the time.

I finally concluded that one of my main areas of discontent was with my home, and for an interior designer, this was a monster of a problem for me. It just no longer fit our lifestyle, and frankly, the constant reminder that this stage of life—raising a family—was over was just too much for me. Our adult kids were not only moving out, they were moving on to locate across the country, which meant we most likely would be visiting them and not vice versa. So what was the point of all these unused rooms that housed all those precious memories and stood constantly empty?

Oh, the house was beautiful, and I had done everything conceivable to it. But unlike my many clients' design projects, no walls could be moved to drastically change this home. We opened up our bedroom and bath a bit, but not enough to really make any big life-changing difference. Trust me when I say there was no way. I can hear some of my clients laughing because, to me, moving a wall or window is just for the good of the design and never a big deal.

In Spite of All Odds…in Spite of All Setbacks…
We Actually Did the Outrageous!

Let me back up a few years to the time before we bought our home we call "Cypress." We were finally seeing an end to years of paying college expenses for all three kids, with our loans coming to an end and our daughter's wedding behind us; but then the bottom fell out for us.

Millions of us Baby Boomers enjoyed the economic boom of the seventies, eighties, and nineties. Regardless of individual social-economic status, this American prosperity morphed into "me and my stuff" materialism. The message was "work hard and your future will be secure," and we Boomers thought this was the way it would always be. Companies were loyal to their employees, and employees were loyal in turn to their employers. Most Boomers expected to work a lifetime career within their company, and it was a big deal to change employers at that time. In over thirty years of my husband Bob working for corporate America, he only changed companies once.

My oh my, how things have changed in America today just in this one area alone. And in just the lifetime of our Boomer generation, we are witnessing a huge change that truly affects all of life in America.

Bob and I know how employment (or lack of it) affects all of life.

"What, Your Job Was Eliminated?"

So, Bob lost his job.

When the other shoe dropped loudly in our life, being

in the category of the unemployed for a hard-working, loyal Baby Boomer like Bob was devastating...especially when we were in our mid-fifties!

"But they told you your job was secure. This was not going to happen to us!"

And there we were; life turned upside down, hit broadside without a warning.

This Was Supposed to Be Our Time to Get Our Finances in Order for Our Boomer Future...Now What?

Suffice it to say that the following years were not only not pretty for us, they were downright ugly! I so understand why many marriages fail in a crisis, whether it is unemployment or sickness or the many other unexpected and forever affecting life crises that, like a thief in the night, come in and rob us of life as we previously knew it.

This is a story within this story with many obstacles and pitfalls too numerous to relate in this writing, but we can say, yes, even proudly, that we did indeed persevere. It was not easy, it was not pretty, but we are intact, and for that fact alone, we give God all the glory.

I will, however, touch on how difficult it is when a very left-brain engineer comes home to work in sales (no less for himself) one room away from my design studio, and me being a very right-brain interior designer. Something just had to give because this, on top of everything else, was most definitely the very last straw of how much this Boomer could and wanted to endure at what was supposed to be our good years.

With much gusto, I say that, fortunately, two years later, Bob was working for a fine company dealing in—of all areas—oil refineries. Well, I must brag that not many know more about oil refineries than my Bob, so it was a match made in heaven...literally.

Spaces

Okay, so one of my serious frustrations was over, and I had my life back for my in-house interior design business, but still the house was just not working.

I teach my students about how eighty percent of our time we live in only twenty percent of our spaces, and that twenty percent should be the ultimate and feed our souls and meet our needs. Well, this certainly wasn't the case for me in our own home.

So, now what?

Enter my artist friend, Joey, who planted the seed of moving into his neighborhood of older homes, with tons of trees and meandering streets, and encouraged us to buy a fixer upper.

Now, I was getting my Boomer fire back for sure! Change, adventure, and possibility were now surging into a hope that I was not going to stay stuck in the mire of staying stuck.

I found in my interior designer's eye a beautiful 1930s home that definitely was a fixer upper. A couple of issues here make this pretty unusual for us late-age Boomers.

The house, first of all, was not for sale, and secondly, to call this home "a fixer upper" was almost a joke; it was so far gone most of our friends said, "Why don't you tear it down and start over?"

Obviously, we did buy this home. But, oh my, the mess, the filth, the dilapidated wiring and plumbing, even the basement foundation. However, I knew that I knew this was to be our future and that it would be a grand future. And you know what? It is grand living in our beloved Cypress home.

Our story of buying our home Cypress, suffice it to say, was my anchor that saved me from drowning into that abyss that I see so many Boomers drowning in. Why do they?

Because so many Boomers accept and believe that this

is all there is, and that there is no way to change things. This is a total kiss of emotional death for sure!

But this is a chapter on Boomer Smart Spaces. So here we go into our world of going on blind faith, literally, without a plan, and moving toward an unknown—but the key here is that we were moving!

Not literally moving, as in only the physical, but we were moving ahead in taking action and not just accepting life's setbacks and that "this is just how it has to be." Are you kidding me? Just suffocate me, for Pete's sake. So we took a huge leap of faith and "moved toward becoming unstuck."

You'll see why next.

Cypress: Our Boomer Smart Home

The saying that "what we tolerate, we will never change" was spot on with how I perceived our family home of thirty years. But I, Mitzi, simply could not tolerate it anymore! And why should our last best rest of our lives be in a home that no longer fit our needs or wants? What would be the harm of selling and moving? And did I say that it simply and absolutely did not meet our needs? Zillions of people do it all the time, so why shouldn't we take the leap of faith to move ourselves into spaces that worked now for this stage of our Boomer life?

This is where I hear some of you readers thinking, "Why, I never heard of anyone being so spoiled that just because she did not like something, she felt she deserved to move." You are darn right! And furthermore, I *do* deserve it. Bob and I have worked hard, and no one has handed us anything on a silver platter. And you also must know that after over forty-five years of marriage, we both continue to work hard to this very day for lots of reasons.

There is a time, I believe, in all Boomers' lives when they must make the decision to "love it or list it," as the HGTV program emphasizes. "If it ain't broke, don't fix it," but if it is broken, well, by golly, get on with your Boomer life and fix it! Why stay in a home that no longer works with outdated everything? And, in most cases, one that is downright not safe for Boomers moving into knee replacement territory, or who are having surgeries, or experiencing myriad other issues that make their present Boomer home nothing more than spaces where an accident is waiting to happen...seriously.

Here is where I ask your forgiveness because I am about to get preachy. Here goes:

Our Spaces Absolutely Affect the Quality of Our Lives

If you could only hear how clients or family respond after I just rearrange furniture or add lighting that makes such a huge differences, you would agree with me that design and our living spaces absolutely affect the quality of our lives.

And furthermore, a good preacher's word, space is not benign. Space not only has the capability to influence in a positive manner, but it most definitely can have a negative influence. Anyone who has ever discovered the profound and lifechanging impact of making their homes full of sanctuary spaces will most certainly exclaim over all the myriad benefits in ways they never considered.

So, in my Boomer mind, I'm saying, "Mitzi, life is short and getter shorter as the years go flying by. Let's get out of these negative-influencing spaces that do not work anymore and into ones that will work for us now and in our future."

And that is exactly what we did when designing our "new" restored, 1930s home, Cypress.

I Believe We Need a Housing Revolution

Yes, you read correctly...we are so far behind in what spaces work for most of us in our present models of homes, that I will only cover the tip of the iceberg here in explaining the whys behind the design of Cypress.

First off, how are we really using our home spaces? Like I always say, eighty percent of our time is spent in only twenty percent of our spaces, so isn't the question that emphatically needs to be asked and answered this: "What should that twenty percent look like?"

Our "twenty-percent spaces" should and need to have at least these top ten qualities:

- The most comfortable and highest-quality furniture.
- Upgraded lighting for all of life's tasks.
- Function, function, function.
- Comfort, comfort, comfort.
- Beauty, beauty, beauty.
- Be filled with life treasures.
- Have luxury items like granite or marble counters.
- Is downsized and free of clutter and meaningless "stuff."
- Have personal sanctuary spaces.
- Controlled sound and privacy.

And this top ten list is just the minimum! If most homeowners actually and realistically evaluated where they spend most of their time in their homes, and use this checklist of what is needed to elevate their lives by the quality of their most-used spaces, Boomer Smart changes could be implemented.

Spaces

What Is So Different in Our Home, Cypress?

Housing Revolution 101—here it comes in our Cypress home with a design that incorporates three living areas or zones:

> Zone #1 Public or entertaining space, guest rooms (first floor).
>
> Zone #2 My interior design studio space (second floor).
>
> Zone #3 Our personal living space (second floor).

Yes, I know, this is all foreign to most people who are thinking, "What in tarnation is she talking about?" Well, remember I said we need a housing revolution, and isn't a revolution about radical change? This is a radical housing design that I have honestly never seen or heard about before, but let me say, it is wonderful! And I can honestly say that Bob and I have only heard sincerely positive comments on our revolutionary design.

So let's walk through Cypress, and I'll explain the why and the how this all works so perfectly, and I must say, so beautifully. If that is boasting, I am guilty as charged, but for heaven's sake, I have been designing homes for over thirty years, so my own home should be beautiful!

The first floor includes the kitchen, living/dining area, mudroom, powder room, two guest bedrooms with a full, barrier-free bathroom, and a morning room off the screened-in porch.

Our Boomer Smart Kitchen

Our kitchen was designed to be the heart of the home where we serve our guests and family with all the atten-

Boomer Smarts, Boomer Power

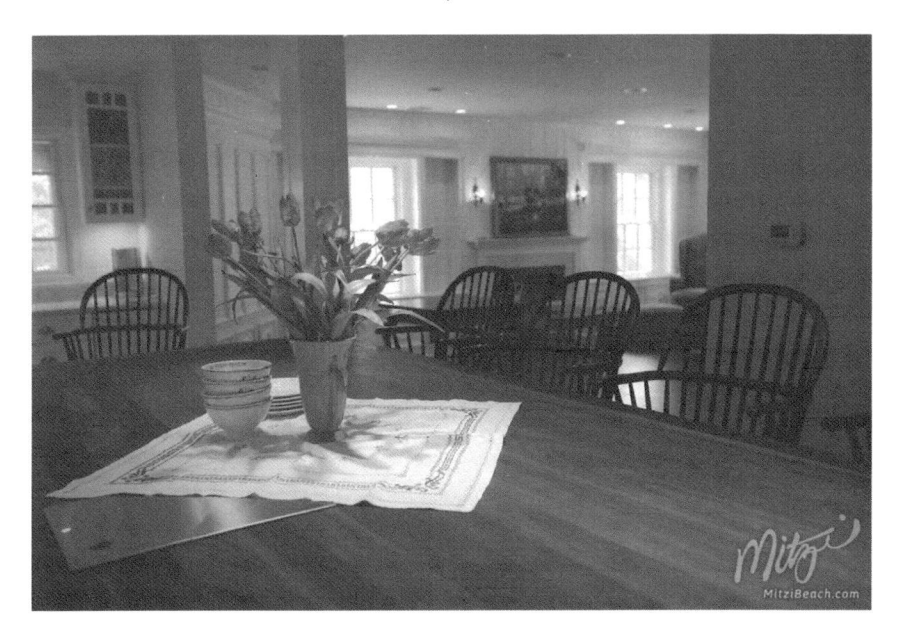

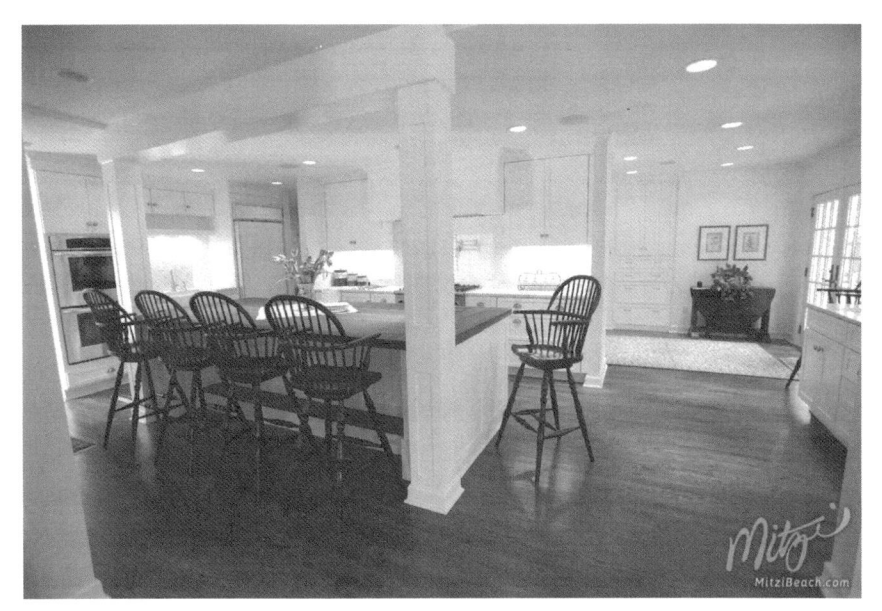

Top: Heart of the Home.
Bottom: Overview of Kitchen.

tion to detail we possibly can include while making our kitchen functional for me, the cook.

To accomplish this goal, first off—and one of my major goals in any kitchen remodel—is to try to keep the island free of major appliances. The reason being is that to use the island for buffets, for dinners, etc., there is just no way to hide the mess from cooking on the stovetop or dishes in the sink. This is my designer opinion, and I could not be more thrilled with our ten-foot long solid walnut island that has been so loved and so used from granddaughters cutting up messy mangos to wedding shower reception buffets and everything in between.

In our family home, we had a 24-square-inch butcher block for an island, and we often commented that it was the most-used inches in our home. Let's see...from a small butcher block to an oversized island...now that's a Boomer Smart upgrade!

Living and Dining Area

I call this open space a fluid area because we can do almost unlimited seating arrangements for various activities and events, whether a sit-down baby shower brunch for thirty ladies or a small dinner party or a cozy area to chat with a friend. It is so much fun for me to entertain in this space that truly was designed to function for these intentional purposes. Plus, Bob and I love sitting here in the winter with the fireplace going and just enjoying the peace and serenity when it is just the two of us. This is why I call this living and dining area a fluid one...it goes with the flow!

The guest rooms are intentionally back out of the way of the living, dining, kitchen, and mudroom areas with the guest rooms having their own dedicated bathroom. As I mentioned, this bathroom is barrier-free, meaning

Boomer Smarts, Boomer Power

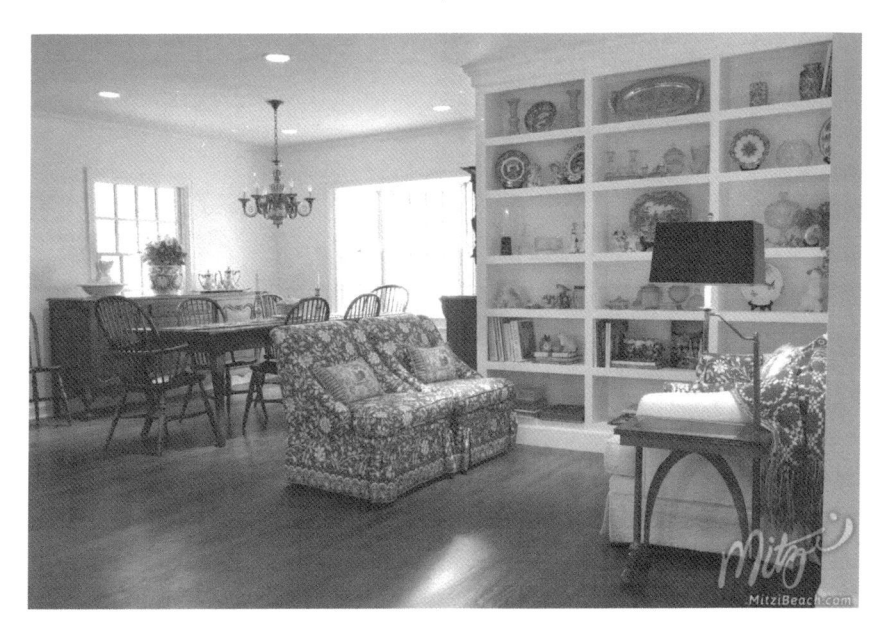

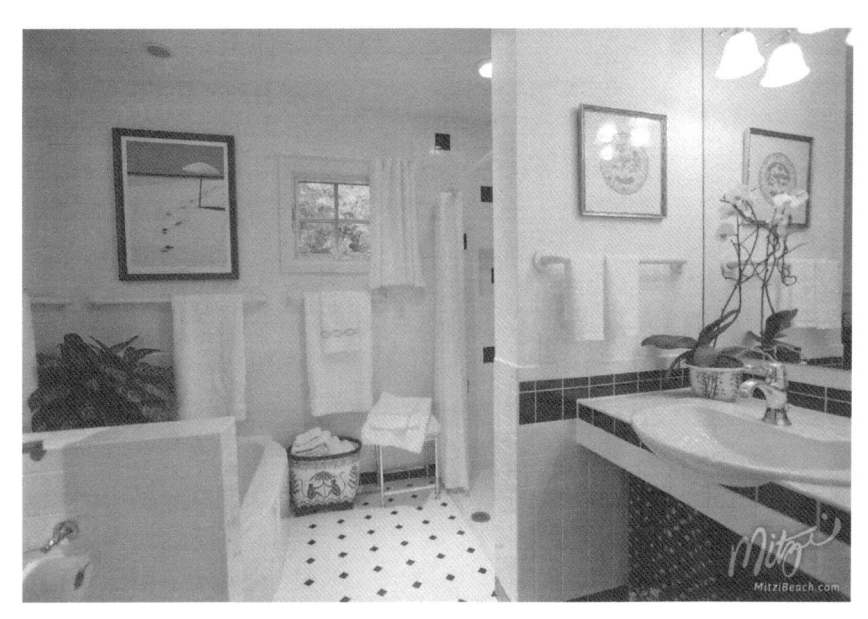

Top: Dining Room Side of Living Area.
Bottom: All Ages Bathroom.

Spaces

there is a shower with no curb; the bath tub, shower, and comfort-height toilet all have grab bars that are white, and I use them for towel bars so no one really thinks this is a hospital-like setting. This bathroom works for my grandchildren as well as elderly parents alike.

My mudroom is probably the key to making the downstairs work like a charm. Included are a walk-in pantry, large coat closet, cleaning closet, counter spaces, sink, and the infamous butcher block from our old home that continues to see lots of "stuff" piled on it as a first pass from the garage. I laugh at myself a lot when I think of me being like Sally Field in the movie *Steel Magnolias* going in her walk-in pantry as she is so upset that her daughter, Julie Roberts, is pregnant with high risks. I loved that movie and I love my walk-in pantry.

The small area that I call the morning room is just a cozy space that separates the kitchen from the private guest bedrooms and bathroom. There is a comfy chair for TV viewing or whatever, and the biggest plus in good weather is that it opens into the screened-in porch...everyone's favorite spot.

Zone #2 is my beloved studio, and I truly mean beloved. Again, there is a large island that is used for absolutely everything in my world, from laying out new design projects, sitting on bar stools working with clients, or sorting the myriad research I did and continue to do for writing on Boomer Life and Design. There are windows on all three sides, so going to work is a lovely experience, especially when it snows, rains, when the leaves change color, during sunsets, sunrises...you get the idea. This studio really is a beloved space to me, which I believe enhances the quality of my work without a doubt.

Zone #3. Okay, this is where everyone is pretty shocked, to say the least. "You what? You live upstairs with your kitchen downstairs? Why didn't you put your master on

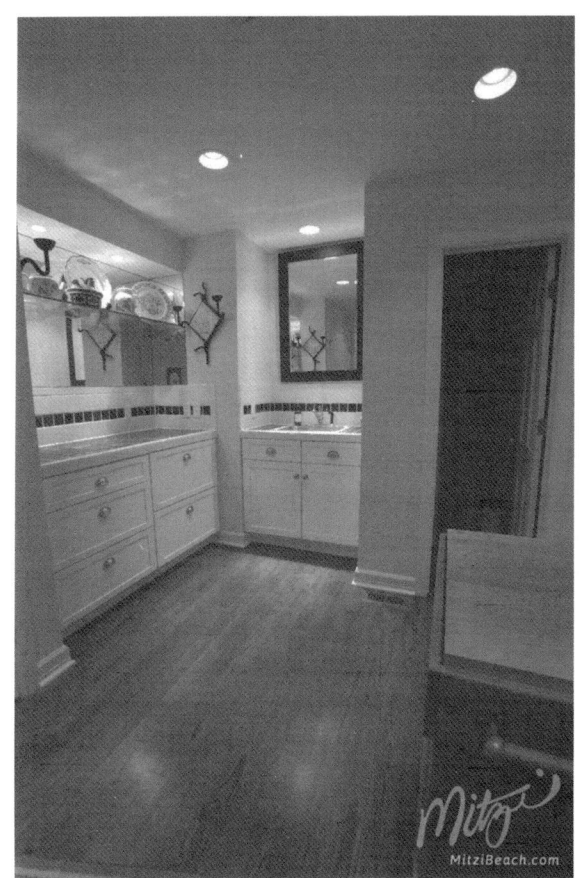

Left: A View of the Mudroom.
Bottom: My Design Studio.

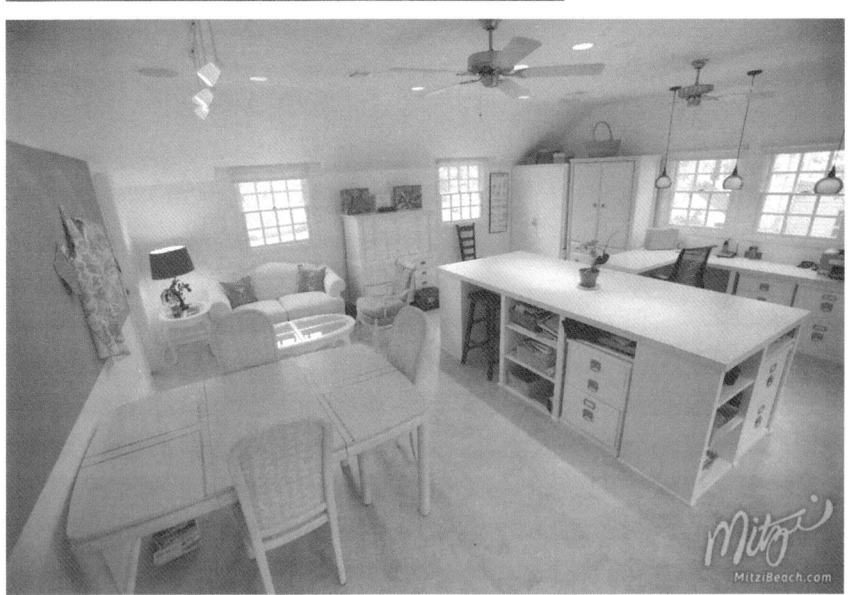

Spaces

the ground floor if you were designing with your future in mind?"

Bob and I just grin, then they see our upstairs apartment or, as we call it, our nest. What cannot be seen, however, is a dedicated space for an elevator if and when it is ever needed.

We have a sitting area with TV, fireplace, mini-kitchen...yes, a mini-kitchen with a cook top and microwave drawer. Our laundry room is off this area, serving also to complete our kitchen needs with a dishwasher drawer, sink, and counter space, along, of course, with tons of storage and a washer and dryer.

Bob's study is off the sitting area, which he loves since for thirty years his desk and all were in a windowless basement. He's now in what we often call his tree house because with window on three sides, it indeed looks like a tree house space.

Then, of course, we have a master suite off our sitting area. It's large enough for two good-size chairs and an ottoman, TV, French doors to a balcony, and again, lots of glazing or windows for lovely natural light and views. Our old home only had small dormer windows, and a big need for Boomers is lots of visual exterior views, which makes such a difference in how we feel...seriously.

My favorite, or one of my zillions of favorite things about Cypress, is our together-but-separate master bathroom! We each have our own water closets and sink areas divided by a small hall with a built-in chest. The shower and tub we share. The bestest part...my area is a dressing-room area with my closet totally open to my bathroom. Yes...I am in love with this design! But you know what? It can be had by lots of Boomers now that Boomers are learning what really is important to them. Many would not like this arrangement, but if the real truth be known, I would be rich if I had a nickel for every

Boomer Smarts, Boomer Power

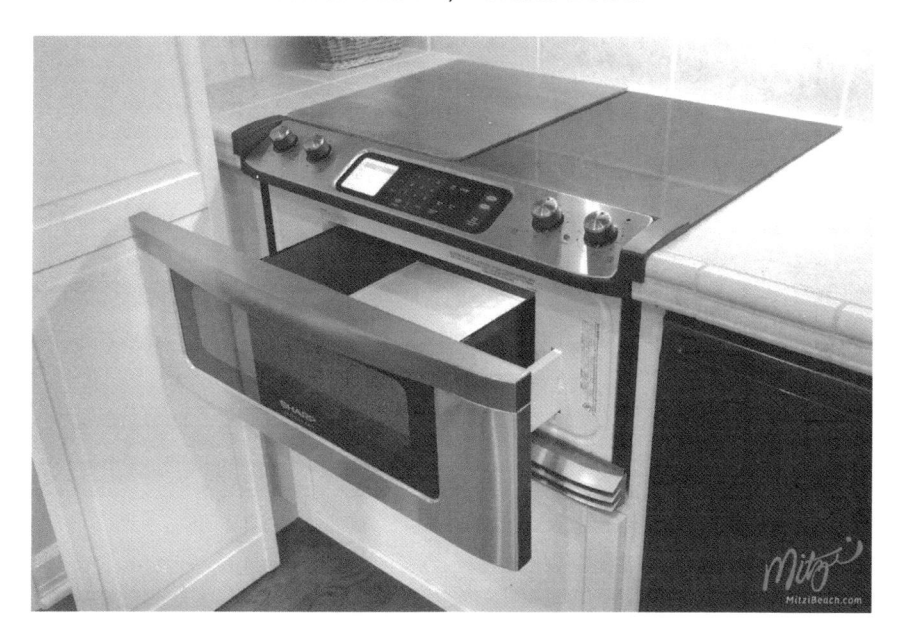

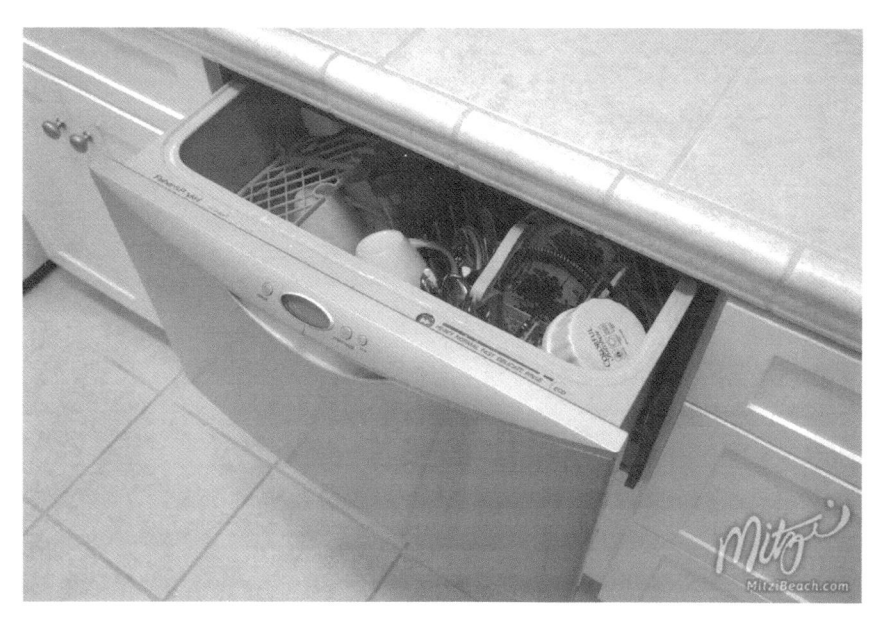

*Top: Microwave Drawer.
Bottom: Dishwasher Drawer.*

Spaces

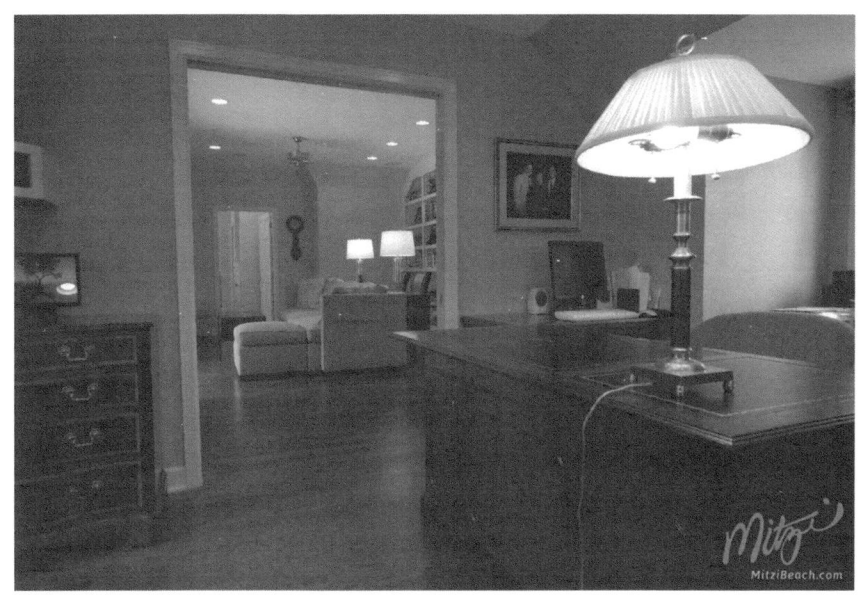

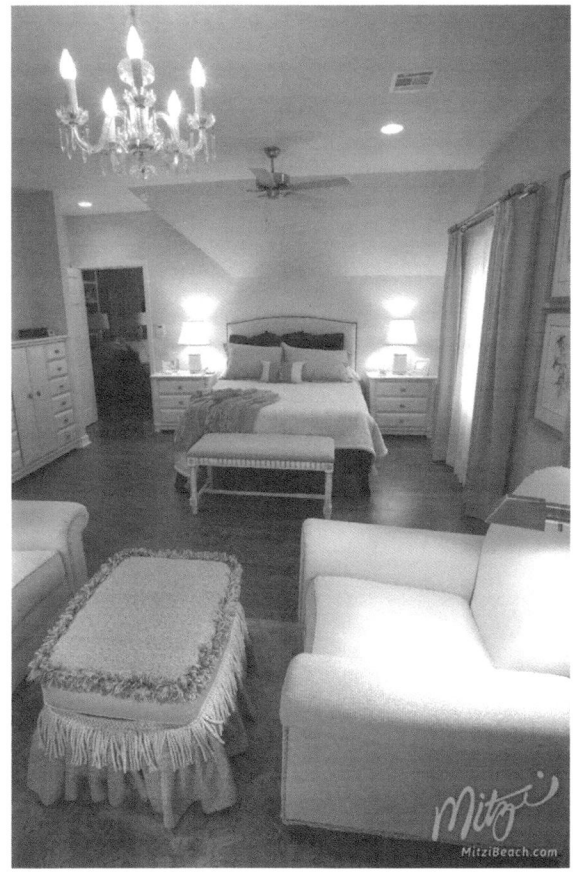

*Above: Bob's Study.
Left: The Master Bedroom.*

33

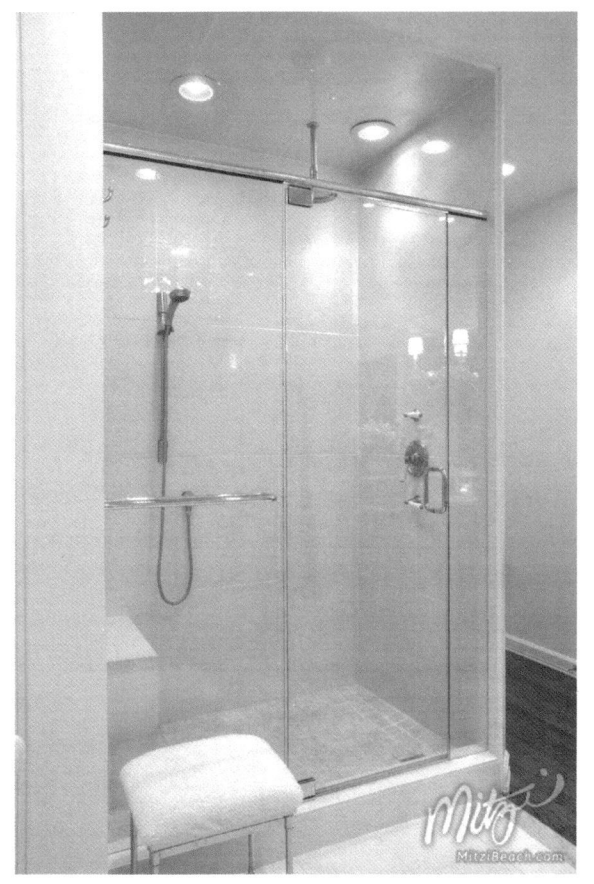

Above: The Master Shower.

woman who says, "Don't tell my husband, but I would love to not share a bathroom with him!" Sorry, guys, it is just a girl thing...or for a lot of girls, anyway.

There you have it. Our version of the beginning of a Boomer housing revolution that has been a long time in coming, but it is indeed on its way. You'll see.

What the Boomer Really Wants in a Home, But Who Is Listening?

"Whether people are fully conscious of this or not, they

actually derive countenance and sustenance from the atmosphere of the things they live in or with."
—Frank Lloyd Wright

Amen to this quote, and my sentiments exactly, as *design affects all of life.*

And I would say without hesitation that poor design affects all of life perhaps even more.

You want proof? Well, falling down stairs because of poor lighting left a friend of mine in a boot cast, which definitely had a negative effect on her life for months. Lighting is a huge and extremely important part of design in our interior spaces. And she said her doctor got up for his nightly bathroom visit in the dark and wham… he broke his foot, too!

On the "bright" side, yes, pun intended, upgrading our lighting is one of the easiest elements for Baby Boomers to accomplish in their homes. I am a lighting fanatic, and I openly admit it even more in this Boomer life stage for myself and my clients. Did you know that at age fifty, we need twice the lighting we did when we were twenty-five?

And yet, *who is listening to even this basic of basics needed for Boomer homes?*

Most Boomers? No.

Most Builders? No.

Most Designers? No.

Okay, before you all stone me, please take note that I said *most*…

Out of the 78 million Boomers, there most certainly are intelligent, courageous, and forward-thinking Boomers, builders, and designers out there buying, building, and designing what Boomers want and what Boomers need in their "Best Rest" or their "Greatest Latest" home, whether remodeling their current home or relocating.

So to those that have the Boomer Smarts to want more knowledge "to live their Boomer wisdom," there is much excitement for what can be an amazing and enriching life experience for Boomers living in homes *designed for their boomer needs and wants.*

Previously, I wrote of the need for a housing revolution that encompasses the reality that American Boomers are changing and so are their housing needs. Now, again and again and again, this is not just about raised toilet seats and grab bars...actually, the politically correct Boomer talk is comfort-height toilets and handrails, just for your information! But seriously, changing our housing spaces is about experiencing a new, better, and more satisfying way of living.

Research in Sage Companion's newsletter says, "A new vision of life at home is close at hand."

How exciting is that? A new vision for our spaces we live in day after day, year after year! I for one am so ready for the pioneer visionaries out there to show us a new revolutionary way of living in our homes—for Boomers of today and seniors of tomorrow. I am excited that new revolutionary models of home design will indeed be the demand of the Boomers with Boomer Smarts.

Already, however, there are most definitely new and extraordinary trends happening. Let's take American demographics, first off, relating how these statistics will affect the coming housing revolution.

A US Census Bureau report released August 27, 2013, shows us that the traditional American household of a married couple with children is quickly becoming the minority rather than the majority of households. I think that this is a startling fact and will certainly affect how we see our homes in the near future.

What really shocked me, actually, was that households with married couples with children shrunk by half between 1970 and 2012, from 40% to 20%. Another shock to me is the number of single Americans living alone, from 17% to 27%. Now, I am not a mathematical genius for sure, but this tells us that over one-quarter of Americans are single and living alone. Recently, however, were statistics that the number of singles in America is over 50% but not counted in the number of singles living in American homes but other forms of housing as condos, etc. If that doesn't get our attention on our changing housing needs, I am not sure what it will take to get the attention of our builders, developers, architects, and designers.

Okay, so things are changing quickly on the American profile, but what does this possibly have to do with any of us? Well, for me, it becomes crystal clear that Boomers, especially, must take stock of what their priorities and needs are in their living spaces for their futures and begin assessing how they will go about meeting these needs and wants.

Boomers do not want the same old floor plans more or less shrunk down and called by another name. Oh no! What research and trend experts tell us will be the most sought-after amenities in Boomer homes are these items or spaces:

- Downsized properties with functional and luxury items.
- Technology home systems now do more than ever, and this of course has just begun to emerge as a must for Boomers. Remotes, keypads, smartphones, or tablets can control or monitor not

only lights, sound systems, temperature control, alarms, sprinkler systems, and window treatments, but also medical information. For example, there is a toilet that can monitor your blood sugar levels...no kidding.
- Laundry mudrooms that multitask for a command-like home center with charging stations, counter space for work, hobbies, pet washing, household storage, and oh, yes...even laundry.
- Master suites that include two sleeping rooms with their own bathroom essentials, such as a water closet and sink, and share shower, tub, and a common sitting area for reading, TV, or personal sanctuary spaces.
- Garages will become safer with zero-clearance entrances or improved entrances with good lighting, handrails, and shelves or cabinets by entrance doors for groceries, etc.
- Kitchens will continue to evolve into the center or heart of the home with user-friendly ergonomic appliances, cabinetry, under-counter lighting, refrigerator, freezer, and dishwasher drawers, easy care everything, pull-out drawers versus doored cabinets, and islands will become ultra important for work, socializing, casual dining, serving, and oh, yes, cooking prep.
- Innovative open space design that brings the outdoors inside, as research and trend watchers convey more visual exterior viewing is not only desired, but is good for our health also by creating calm and allowing us to experience nature.
- Easy-care everything, including flooring materials, furniture, counters, etc.
- Outdoor patio with privacy and optional gardening space.

- Outdoor kitchens.
- Entertaining spaces are very important, with storage for functional equipment, serving, and with multi-task furniture to serve as work areas or entertaining, as in more casual tables and seating that also can serve Thanksgiving dinner using Grandma's china.
- Open-space designed homes will be reevaluated to include multitasking activities like computer work areas along with TV viewing for family and guests.
- Personal sanctuary spaces will be common as Boomers' lives continue to be or get busier whether they are retired or not.
- Upgraded lighting and lighting systems will become the norm, especially among single women, for security inside and out.
- "Storage, storage, storage" is the cry of the Boomer; even though downsizing, they want what they want when they want it.
- Luxury bathroom items like steam showers, heated-tile flooring, large sauna-type showers, therapeutic bathtubs to soothe all aches and pains away and not simply a Jacuzzi tub, TV and sound systems, cabinetry with drawers versus doored cabinetry for easy use, luxury tiles and counter materials, high-end fixtures, and, of course, upgraded lighting everywhere, including sensors to turn on and off during those nighttime trips to the bathroom.
- Doorways to be a minimum of 32 inches and even 36 inches. Hallways four-feet wide. Stairs with handrails on both sides and three-way switches.

These are not unrealistic goals for our homes of the future. So much of our financial costs in our homes are on items we no longer care about or rooms we no longer use or need. By truly evaluating exactly what is important and eliminating those things that are not, many of these housing trends will be affordable to many Boomers. Instead of taking the allotted "pot of money" and spreading it throughout the home, take the same amount of money and use it for what Boomers truly want and need. The same amount of money is spent but on items and rooms that are for the Boomer of today and not merely more of the same old tired floorplans.

Our Boomer spaces of the future will be different, but they will be better for those Boomers equipped with the Boomer Smarts to even know what to ask for and then go after it. These Boomer homes will be so beyond the typical standard downsized home. You'll see.

Bonus List for the Really Smart Boomer

And now for those Boomers that are so, so smart they are actually going to "live their wisdom" by incorporating upgrades and products to make their homes not only more convenient, but safer. This list is for you.

- Contrasting color for bottom steps or floor areas where tripping could be an issue.
- Slip-resistant bathroom surfaces.
- Additional lighting everywhere.
- Laundry on the first floor by master bedroom, or an upstairs laundry space.
- Minimal number of throw rugs and area rugs (use double-sided tape).
- Master and full bath on first floor or dedicated spacing to accommodate an elevator if needed.
- Doors with 32- to 36-inch openings to accommodate walkers, wheelchairs.

- Handrails on both sides of stairways.
- Appliances and cabinetry to meet ergonomic conveniences.
- Different heights for kitchen counters.
- Short-pile carpeting or hard-surface flooring.
- Lever door and fixture handles (instead of knobs).
- Comfort-height toilets and grab bars in bathrooms.
- Zero clearance or no curb for shower.
- Eliminate shower/tub combinations for master bath.
- Showers with sit-down bench and hand-held shower; a second showerhead option.
- Garage entry to house with handrail, landing, lighting.
- Less furniture and traffic patterns free from clutter.
- Efficient storage spaces, even in garages.
- Windows that open easily.
- Porch or private patio.
- Bigger bathrooms.
- Energy-efficient HVAC and appliances.
- Security systems and Smart Home Technology systems.

These added adjustments, remodeling and safety tips, and convenience and ergonomic suggestions for Boomer homes will indeed prepare Boomers to live the best years of their lives in their own homes, maintaining the best of life for the rest of life. You'll see.

Boomer Smart Stories

Cindy Carnahan
The Carnahan Group
www.TheCarnahanGroup.com

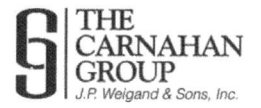

THE CARNAHAN GROUP
J.P. Weigand & Sons, Inc.

Mitzi: You cannot sell what is not on the market. You and I discussed that recently. So, the first question is: Do you believe like I do, that we need a housing revolution? If so, what are you not seeing in the homes you sell?

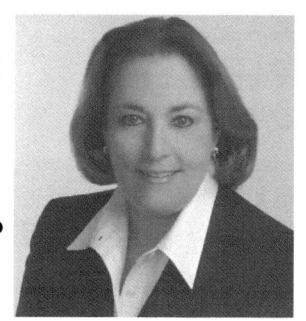

Cindy: Well, Wichita is a small market, as we all know. So, we certainly don't have a lot of the product that is available in larger markets. I'm not saying high-rise but luxury high-rise apartment living, which I think there is a demand for from Baby Boomers who would like to see a high-rise that offers amenities and security and ease of living that we're seeing in the patio homes. But there's another step, I think, between patio home and the home, if you will, and that would be the high-rise luxury apartment type, and even a cooperative where you could own your own apartment. We aren't seeing it here, but I'm sure they're seeing it in other areas of the country.

Mitzi: Definitely.

Cindy: That is something that we could use, but my understanding is that the infrastructure is so expensive to build that that's why there's no risk being taken on that type of construction. New construction, all in all—there isn't any risk out there much. No new developments truly have come online. Maybe a couple, but the banks are reticent to jump back into that pool of builders, and they're still feeling the losses that they suffered during the downturn.

So, we're not seeing a lot of new construction. I am feeling like the Baby Boomers want a lot less square footage than these patio homes have, and a lot higher-quality finishes. As a result, the Baby Boomers feel compelled to either stay where they are longer than they should, or they move on to the patio home, and they have the finished basements that they don't even use.

Mitzi: Right.

Cindy: That's kind of what I'm seeing that's not out there.

Mitzi: Okay. So, really, then, it's interesting. I mean, I'm not putting words in your mouth, of course, but that reinforces what my belief is—that we do indeed need a housing revolution. There's essentially a huge Baby Boomer needs and wants gap in Boomer housing not being built. So, it is going to be very interesting.

What my clients tell me they're after is luxury items, and the latest and greatest finishes. They want the beautiful surfaces and fixtures in their bathroom and kitchen and not rooms they will never use. No, they're after something new and different in home space planning.

So, what is the biggest mistake you see your Boomer clients making in evaluating their new home purchases?

Cindy: Well, all buyers do this: they go out to purchase what they don't have and they forget about the things they love that they do have. And everybody does that. Everybody does that across the board, and then they get there and they go, "But I used to have a..." "And I don't have..."

So, you know, they want what they don't have but they forget about the things that they love that they do currently have.

Mitzi: Okay, if you could advise and/or influence your Boomer clients, what is your number-one tip? What should they be looking for? And it does not need to be the number one, just—you already answered with the mistakes about forgetting what they had in the past, just looking for the new and—

Cindy: Right. I would say they still need to look for location. They need to seek out privacy if they can.

Mitzi: This is so true. Well, thank you, Cindy. I just wanted your take on this and get your Boomer thoughts, and I think one of the biggest takeaways I have in speaking with you is the high-rise, that in between that we don't have.

But even when we have areas that have patio homes, we're not seeing many builders that would take one or two lots and make a community center.

And that's what people have in other cities that I have visited and studied.

Even in this high-rise model, there is often a community center where people do dinners or classes or have functions or what not. It's about community and it's about connecting. And I'm seeing that as a huge void that we don't have in our areas here.

Cindy: I'm sure that's true. And with the churches becoming less and less important...but I see exactly what you're saying too, yeah.

Mitzi: People are lonely and disconnected often as Boomers. They want to connect but they don't know how, especially Baby Boomers that don't have any kids in school anymore. It's like, how do they get out there in the community? Cindy, thank you so much. I appreciate it.

Kelly Kole
Kandrac Kole Interiors
www.Kandrac-Kole.com

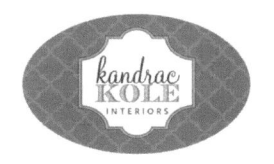

Mitzi: What is your perspective—being a designer, of course, and seeing myriad clients and homes—what is your perspective on whether Boomers have considered their future when they're designing their homes? We're not talking about just raised toilet seats and grab bars. But, overall, what are you seeing in this huge Boomer market that we're researching, all 78 million of us?

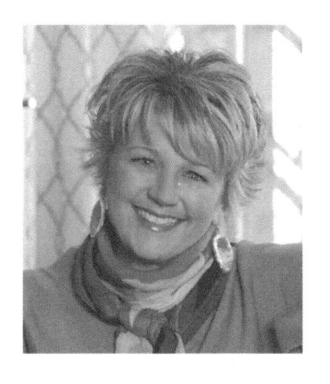

There's going to be—seeing the prediction, it's like a tsunami coming and we're not prepared. And so, that's where we come in as designers, along with others, of course, but we have the opportunity, the responsibility, and the privilege to influence their lives greatly.

Kelly: Yes.

Mitzi: So, my first question to you is, in designing your client's home, your philosophy states function as a goal. Your Boomer clients, which probably are most of them, who would be anyone born from 1946 to 1964. So, the oldest are sixty-seven and the youngest are fifty. Do most of your clients fall into that range?

Kelly: We are probably more in the forty to sixty range, but definitely, a big handful of Boomers for sure.

Mitzi: And that Boomer is actually right where, really, the market void is from the vendors, suppliers, etc. This is what has not been tapped into, that is the core of where a lot of the wealthiest Americans are age wise. But anyway, since a lot of your clients fall into this age group, the Boomer, do you see any of them thinking ahead as far as planning their spaces when you're involved with their projects?

Kelly: No, I don't see them planning ahead. I see us planning ahead, so lucky for them that they have called us to design their home.

But for them, no. I think it's more they don't know what's available, and they aren't thinking ahead to how aesthetics and function can really mix. And so, they're relying on us for that universal design because it probably hasn't even occurred to them. Especially if they don't have any physical disabilities at that particular time, like my parents.

My parents just moved into a new house in Upstate New York. And really, they're very, very active and they're always on the go, and it wasn't until my mom had her hip replaced six months ago that all of a sudden for the very first time, my mom said to me, "I have never been in a hospital since I had you girls." And I'm forty-five, so, she had never thought about, "Oh, my gosh, you know, maybe my traffic patterns in my rooms need to be a little bit wider or my sofa needs to be a little bit stiffer because it's harder for me to get up out of it right now." Things like that. So, I don't think that our clients are necessarily planning ahead like they should.

Mitzi: I could not agree with you more. It's just interesting gathering these facts because I'm privileged to have you—and the other interviewees who live all over the country. So just to be able to hear what is going on in various places, it's going to be really helpful.

But what I'm hearing, Kelly, is basically you're saying that until there's a real need, the light bulb doesn't go on, i.e, the designer or the—we very rarely see it from the builder part and, sadly, not really even from the architect at this point. We designers are really the ones that are in the clients' personal lives and spaces. We learn how they're going to function. I don't know if you agree with that or not, but—

Kelly: Oh, yes, one hundred percent.

Mitzi: We get a relationship built. We know how they live. You've already given some examples of what to consider when you were talking about wider hallways and traffic patterns, and they're excellent.

Are there some other things that you would suggest for your clients—who are mostly in the forty to sixty age range, I think you said—but that would be palatable to them, that you could come in through the backdoor. What kind of things would you suggest that they consider?

Kelly: Well, you know, it's funny because when I was thinking about your questions and how I would answer them, it occurred to me that really we are making the same decisions design-wise for my older clients as I am my younger clients because I think that in this day and age, everybody is looking for function and practicality and comfort. So, for example, I have a couple who are in their early forties that we just designed for, and they wanted a dual reclining loveseat for their family room. Well, we automatically back motorized reclining when we're doing, you know, motion furniture. It's always motorized, which is so much easier for everybody. Nobody wants to have to reach down to the seat and grab that lever and pull. You might not have that strength or that dexterity as you get older, but when you're younger, you don't want to deal with it either. Or, for example, we just finished a kitchen renovation, and I am a big fan of the pull-out drawer microwave.

Mitzi: I have one. I love it.

Kelly: Who wants to do all that bending or reaching when you don't have to today with the countertops that are higher? It's right there. Also, for example, hard wood. Everybody wants hard wood these days. And that's so much easier for mobility of wheel chairs or that kind of thing. Tripping is a big issue.

Mitzi: But just allergy issues and all the things associated with fibers and dust mites, etc.

Kelly: We do address these issues. That's funny that you say that because we do so much hypoallergenic furniture these days. No down, just looking for all those eco-friendly materials that are now available.

People are just figuring that out now. The other thing with furniture is we're finding—and this is with our younger clients' house—is wow, it's just, if you have had back issues or a bad back or like me, our knees are shot from years of running in tennis, we are specifying custom sofas. So, for example, the back cushion might be TempurPedic, but the seat cushion is a little stiffer so it's easier to get out of.

Mitzi: That's awesome.

Kelly: But our clients would never even know that existed because they can't get that in a retail market.

Mitzi: Right, for sure, unless working with someone like yourself in the know of what can be done.

Kelly: So, when we're asking all those function questions, "Do you lay down?" "Do you sit down?" "Do you have your feet up?" "What is your lifestyle—do you entertain a lot?" "What are your family members like?" We just had a new client who said, "My in-laws come to visit all the time, and to be honest, they're extremely overweight. And so it's hard for them to get out of chairs." And so we are really cognizant about that when we're sourcing the chairs.

Mitzi: Okay. Excellent. Kelly, you are way ahead of most designers. I'm very impressed. How do you see yourself in your personal housing for meeting your future needs—have you already done things, Kelly, or what are you enjoying now that works for you, or what things would you like to tweak?

Tell me about yourself personally, if you care to share that, what works for you in your house. What you would like to change for this stage of your life?

Kelly: Well, I would say that as my skill and experience has grown as an interior designer, I've realized that I can make a room beautiful with my eyes shut. But it doesn't necessarily mean that that space has any meaning to me. So, you know, a lot of these Boomers are, as they say, aging in place. They're staying put where they are. They're not necessarily running to a nursing home, but are not moving yet either. They're trying to stay at home as long as they can. And so, for me, this is the same for how we deal with our clients. We're constantly looking for how we can preserve memories, how we can design around something special, how we can custom-make something special. We do a lot of photo galleries where we will take a huge pile of photographs from a client and we will scan them and turn them black and white—

Mitzi: I saw that on your blog. I saw your design partner, Joann, doing this very thing.

Kelly: Yes. We do a lot of those. And they're not — it's not an inexpensive way to decorate a wall, but it brings tears to our clients.

Mitzi: Yes, and that's what I've been spending a lot of time doing for my own home. It's just making sure that if I'm going to invest in something, it's something that is going to stick with me for a long time. I'm kind of over just, you know, running out real quick and buying something pretty. Well, Joann posted something recently where she said that it's all about our treasures or important items or something like that, and I commented on my artist friend Joey, who called things for things' sake…that stuff…junk on parade. Isn't that what you're talking about, junk on parade?

Kelly: Uh huh.

Mitzi: And that's the way I feel about it. I'm just not out to impress anyone at this stage of life. We don't just go out and purchase to purchase. It needs to be something that involves them or they're…they're involved in doing it. So, that's an excellent point.
　So, what you're doing is you're trying to bring meaning into your home that is more personal.

Kelly: Yeah, I want things to have a story, even if they're not necessarily the origin of that item, but I can remember, "Oh, that was the day that I went to lunch with my best friend and we stopped at that random antique store and I saw that weird bench and I just bought it because I loved it. And I didn't know what I was going to do with it and I ended up, you know, redoing it and…" Those kinds of things, that I didn't run out to the local department store to get.
　And that's really the main philosophy that we've used for our clients. I mean, we're always rummaging through attics and basements and bringing out things that our clients will say, "Oh, that old thing? I love that. It was my great aunt's that she rocked every baby in, but it's so old now." And we're like, "Oh, no, no. We are going to restore this and we're going to put this smack-dab in the middle of your home room."

Mitzi: I love it. Yes, exactly, Kelly. Before I forget, how old is your mother that had the hip replacement?

Kelly: My mom is seventy.

Mitzi: Okay. So, she's been really healthy up until then. That's awesome. So, in your own home with your family—from what I gather reading your blogs and what not, I think your girls are in college—

Kelly: Yes, uh huh.

Mitzi: So now your future master plan. Are you thinking differently about what your personal interior space is going to be? Staying in your present home or moving? Are you thinking of remodeling your spaces to be the ultimate master suite and new spaces and whatnot, or do you see leaving it?

Kelly: Leaving it for sure.

Mitzi: Okay.

Kelly: For me, personally, I want to downsize. I want something small and perfect in every way.

Mitzi: Love that.

Kelly: You know, I've just gotten to a point in my life where I like material things and I like beautiful thing but I don't need a lot of them. So if I could just have a little cottage with a tiny little perfect backyard and everything that I care about, you know, done beautifully, that's all I want.

Mitzi: I can see it, Kelly.

Kelly: My house now, it's just too—and it's not even big. It's like 3800 square feet. It's just too big—I don't need all that.

Mitzi: Right, right. I hear you. That's a beautiful thing. I can see that cottage and all that goes with it. There's no doubt. It's a matter of time, and you will have that perfect place.

Kelly: You give me a really beautiful front porch and two rocking chairs and a beautiful garden, and I'm happy. That's exactly what I want.

Mitzi: What is the biggest mistake you see your Boomer clients, your clients making in their home? I know they have you and Joann, but even so, is there any obstacle that you find with your design business that is just a constant challenge of what people are either fighting you on or not getting or—

Kelly: No, I think we're blessed that our clients trust us implicitly, so we don't argue much with them, but what we try to do, especially with this group, is walk into spaces and say, "Okay, this room has been a dining room forever. You use it twice a year. Do you want it to be something different?" You know, reevaluating every space so that it maximizes for how they live today or how they will live in the future.

For example, these Boomers are going to work a lot longer than the previous generation. So, they can be working into their sixties. And so does that living room that you never use need to become your home office on the first floor that you can access easier without stairs? Or the kids are all gone. Do you have to have four bedrooms? Can one of them be a music room? A reading room? A hobby room? An arts and crafts room? Something that will make you happy doing what you love as you get older when maybe you can't leave the house as much as you used to.

Mitzi: Excellent.

Kelly: Those kinds of things. So, I would say probably the one mistake would be not really thinking outside the box as to "how can I re-function my space?"

Mitzi: Okay, I love it. In your area, are you seeing home design that is a cut above, or do you see your builders and developers recognizing this age of the Baby Boomers and their need of not just another patio home that may just be a smaller version of homes that are already out there? Are they getting it? Are you seeing a change in home designs in your area for this age group?

Kelly: I'm not seeing a change. Well, let me say that Atlanta is so over-saturated and was hit so hard by the recession that we haven't had a big surge of construction in the last eight years. But the only time that I'm really seeing the things that you and I are talking about is when it's in an assisted living or an older community that's marketed towards older folks. In the general homes that are being built for the public, I do not see specific things like lowered outlets and bigger windows for better lighting and thermostats at a certain height and doorknobs that are levers and not round knobs, and all those things for when your mobility and dexterity are going. It affects you. So, no, I don't see that.

Mitzi: Well, you can tell by what the questions were and how you're answering them and what you're seeing and doing in your design business that this is going to be a huge movement, a huge shift in the not-too-distant future.

Kelly: And I think it also points very, very strongly at

the value of an interior designer who is educated and full of resources for this generation.

Mitzi: Excellent, Kelly. I could talk to you all day. You are just an inspiration to us all. I'm thrilled to have this little slice of time with you. Thank you so much.

Kelly: Oh, good. Well, I'm so happy to help you. And you know, for these people, I think of my parents. You don't know what you don't know, and so if you don't have a person, an interior designer or somebody in front of you saying, "You know what? What if we cut out that closet and make an elevator," how would you even know? How do you even think of that if you don't know what you don't know?

Mitzi: That's exactly correct! And that's the whole premise of the Boomer Smarts goals—to motivate and inspire this whole movement. We need outward-thinking, progressive-thinking designers like you and Joann because it's amazingly sad to still say how many builders, designers, and architects are just very satisfied with doing things the way they've always done them. And you and I push that proverbial envelope to be just better and higher and different and smarter that I'm proud to say that there is just a whole lot of pride in our industry that says, in effect, don't mess with Texas. It's like we already know and we are doing just fine, thank you. So, it's about, again, the savvy Baby Boomer builders, architects, designers, for those that have ears to hear, eyes to see, and are going to live a very cool way of life. Those are our people and my mission is not everybody. My mission is to just start this whole conversation and dialogue and see where we go with it. So, thank you again, Kelly.

Geri Higgins
Portfolio Kitchen & Home
www.portfolio-home.com

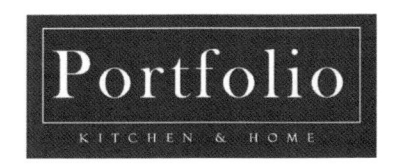

Mitzi: In my humble opinion, I believe we need a housing revolution to meet the demanding and changing needs of this huge Boomer demographic—and not just aging in place, but functional designing, period. If you agree, please share what you are not seeing in homes you design.

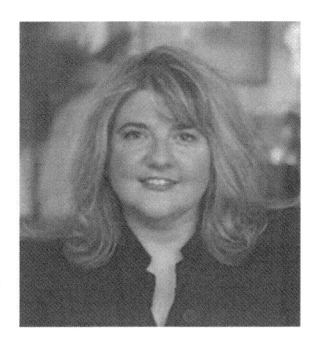

Geri: First of all, what I'm not seeing is really a master plan, a plan for now but definitely a plan for later on. And one that celebrates not only your signature style but more importantly your signature lifestyle. And lifestyle touches all of the assets—in what we do, how we do it. It's how we're going to succeed in the later years.

This is a critically important issue, that you should have a master plan, and it's very, very important when you are going through this design process to not only celebrate your style but your lifestyle, to really kind of break down who you are, what you want, and the what ifs. Be sure that you're prepared for all of it.

So, a master plan is really more of a celebration of just everything that is going to happen in life. Design is usually only focused on style, not lifestyle. Like, what are the things that we do, how do we do them, how are we to progress, what can we deal with in our life through the design process, how can we elevate it and celebrate it and optimize it even when life changes, our body changes, time changes.

Mitzi: Excellent point and exactly right on for truly using and doing design as it is meant to be—all inclusive in all of life, as you said so succinctly, Geri.

On to question two. What would be at the top of your list as to what Boomers should be doing or looking for in their home remodeling or future home?

Geri: Smart choices that are super attractive, but ones that address life's major challenges, okay? So, design to celebrate, like hobbies or interests or how to optimize and elevate one's lifestyle for the later years.

So, the important thing is to embrace lifestyle, design for celebrating your life no matter what your life's condition, and when it comes to body function, the keywords are ergonomics, usability, and functionality. And so, we can get in to how that can work in different parts with the house. For example, in the kitchen. When you're utilizing drawers in the kitchen design, they are very, very attractive. It's more attractive than doors because it looks more furniture-like, but it also has a second benefit, and that second benefit is fantastic for visibility, for usability, and great for body function.

So, something that you're designing today that might be very forward in a design way, and in a design trend, or just making a strong aesthetic is actually something that's going to work for you in later years. So, that's an important thing. Also, things like dishwashing drawers. Well, those are wonderful to have and especially when they're integrated and hidden in your furniture like cabinets. It's wonderful because it's also easy to access and it's a drawer so it's higher up. So it's easier to load.

That's another way to say that something that is attractive now is highly functional later. Also, appliances, when you're thinking about appliances and placement, not only do you want to think about placement for usability. For example, ovens that are stuck in the wall but also the visibility of the controls of those appliances that you're buying now just to make sure that there's wording and numbers that are easy to read.

Mitzi: Exactly right again, Geri. My son-in-law, a malpractice attorney and obviously very smart, was staring at the door of their new refrigerator and asking, how do I get a glass of water out of here? We can do better!

Geri: Yes, I am on the Thermador design team, and we evaluate that very thing along with product design.
So now bathrooms: You need to think about right now how it's really a beautiful statement to have a floor that just seamlessly connects to your shower. And to have bright open bathrooms with glass that goes from the floor to ceiling.
Well, how will that function later on in life? Well, it would be nice to have it barrier-free. So, no curb between the floor and the shower, so that it's one continuous piece. So, no matter what, you can have access into that shower. Also, think about having a bench in the shower and the extra hand-held shower unit that's next to the bench, which is really spa-like because you can use it now for shaving and other things but later on, if there's a medical reason, you can sit on that bench and utilize that shower, that hand-held shower.

Mitzi: Most definitely these elements are for Boomers now, not just in their futures as you are relating. How many Boomers are having knee and hip replacements and cannot use their own bathrooms? We would be shocked to know.

Question number three: what is the biggest mistake you observe Boomer clients making in their design decisions when they don't heed your advice?

Geri: I think failing to make a plan is critical because no matter what the design process is going to cost, a certain amount of money, but for a little bit more money and a little bit more time in planning, you can have really an excellent, future game plan now, a design that will function not only now but in later years.

So, I think that the biggest problem is people just not addressing that design can be functional and more as you move into the next life stages.

Mitzi: Yes, and sadly, Geri, with the exception of those wanting more out of their homes and who are seeking designers that have the knowledge and experience to make it happen, many projects fail in their design potential to truly change lives. Question number four, in your own personal living spaces, what do you love and why? What would you do differently, if anything?

Geri: I love my casual living space—I have a formal Georgian—but I really utilize my casual living space, which includes my kitchen, casual dining, and conversation areas, making this area the heart of my home. And usually in later years, no matter what size the home is, it's important to have that space that you can absolutely celebrate life in no matter the life stage.

I think also that that kind of area is very functional. In design for homes in the future, the open floor plan really works very well, because usually you're going to be spending most of your time there and it's more part of the house. Usually it's between the kitchen, informal dining, and your casual gathering place. So, that's all open. That works very well. Also incorporating washers and dryers, instead of having them in the basement, to have them part of your master en suite. It's more convenient in the future, but it's also just a lovely kind of empowering action for now. I've made sure I had a washer and dryer off of my master suite, not wanting to be going up and down the stairs and later on in life, which I think this focuses about, is to make sure you can celebrate your life in a biggest way easily. And so, most definitely, I think that that's an empowering change, having your washer and dryer also in your master bedroom instead of going down to a basement or laundry room off the garage when you're older.

Mitzi: Absolutely, or even now or even at any age, right? So last question. What, if anything, would you do differently in your own home?

Geri: I'm in the process of redoing my master bath, and it's the little things that we talked about that I'm actually implementing. I'm doing it for the style part of it, but also to be functional, so if I decide to live in this house forever and ever, I'll be able to.

Mitzi: Well, Geri, your insight has been extremely valuable to all Boomers out there who truly want the best out of design, which you have stated emphatically celebrates life at all stages. This can only be accomplished by a thought-out and guided master plan that designs for the now of life and the future of life.

No wonder you are so successful! Thank you for your time.

Chapter 2
Mindsets

Make Up Thy Boomer Mind to Be Boomer Smart

Ninety percent of the game is half mental.
—Yogi Berra

Changed my mind.
Out of my mind.
A woman has a right to change her mind.
Make up your mind.
Keep in mind.

Why a chapter each on mindsets and attitudes?

Well, as the great late Satchel Paige said, "Age is mind over matter; if you don't mind, it doesn't matter."

A mindset and an attitude are very much the same, but for our purposes of understanding how to break down strongholds or paradigms, or mindsets, an entire chapter is devoted to "making up our minds" to age better and smarter, i.e., to equip ourselves with Boomer Smarts.

What does a Boomer with a Boomer Smart mindset look like?

One with a Boomer Smart mindset is not naïve, but is

able to discern what is happening right now in America and can acknowledge and accept the fact that personal changes are immensely critical to prepare for our futures.

BOOMERS BEWARE!

Even though I am a research guru on Boomer trends and current happenings, I was totally shocked—like kicked-in-the-stomach shocked—when I had my first refusal to be seen by a doctor simply because I was on Medicare!

I had wanted to get another opinion on a physical issue, so I called this doctor's office to make an appointment. The first question from the receptionist was not my name or my age or even my reason for wanting an appointment. No. It was, "What kind of insurance do you have?"

When I replied that my primary insurance was Medicare (government mandated for anyone sixty-five and older) with supplemental Blue Cross and Blue Shield, her brisk response was, "We do not take Medicare patients."

Wow. Just like that, I had been labeled and refused! Now, I am blessed with excellent health and have worked hard to maintain my health, so I am not one to abuse the medical system.

But, and this is a huge "but," this is a wake-up call to ALL BOOMERS!

Things are changing in America, and in order to prepare for our futures, action is required. A different MINDSET is critically needed for those who assume our government will continue to take care of our physical needs, through either Medicare or Social Security.

This simply is not the case anymore in America, and yet a prevalent MINDSET prevails either consciously or

Mindsets

unconsciously that our physical needs will somehow be taken care of...a totally unsubstantiated MINDSET based on what?

Sadly, I believe that Americans today are vastly naive regarding current happenings in changing government policy and health care. But even if it were the same as our parents had, who wants to live long but live taking tons of meds and having one medical issue after another?

And not only is American health care changing, but the number of Boomers who will someday be in need of home modifications to function safely within their own spaces is rising.

A silver tsunami is absolutely happening that is affecting the huge numbers of Americans entering our social systems. Every day, 12,500 Americans turn fifty years old. And by 2020, 75 million Americans will be over sixty! This is thirty-four percent more than in 2012.

> *It is staggering how unprepared we are.*
> —Ken Dychtwald
> Age Wave

Do the math. Where will all these Boomers live? With single-parent families now making up over half of all families, what financial and lifestyle preparation is being done to prepare for these single adults' future living spaces?

Yes, my fellow and beloved Boomers, change is indeed upon us. But those of us with Boomer Smarts will recognize what is happening and start now TO CHANGE

OUR MINDSETS ON OUR OWN AGING AND GET REAL REALITY ABOUT WHAT IS AHEAD.

My heart truly hurts as I observe and hear so many Boomers being so nonchalant regarding their own situations. Thus, at the risk of being the doomsayer, I am willing to take that risk for the sake of enlightening those who will hear this wake-up call.

However, for those who will hear and develop a new Boomer mindset, mental doors will open to obtain Boomer knowledge. And with their Boomer knowledge, they will gain Boomer wisdom, which will lead to Boomer understanding and then..."Aha!" moments happen as they live in their wisdom in the ultimate Boomer Power.

This, my fellow Boomer, is the ultimate goal of Boomer Smarts. For each of us Boomers, aging brings new life events as our children grow up, as we become empty nesters in homes that no longer meet our needs, as we launch adult children, organize their weddings, and receive daughter- or son-in-laws; physical needs change, careers are changed or lost, and caring for and loving grandchildren and aging parents take a priority. Whew! This is only part of all these life stages and changes.

Our New Mindset

So now, let me tell you about our life changes and Cypress, our 1930s home that we restored in our late fifties, or I should say "rescued" from a tear down. Talk about gaining and receiving a new MINDSET, for Pete's sake! Everyone, and I mean *everyone*, thought we were "out of our ever-loving minds."

Boomers are those born from 1946 to 1964, and for older Boomers, the reality of corporate downsizing, recession, and business closings has been very frightening, because at our age there is not enough time left to reposition ourselves financially for retirement.

My husband Bob was a corporate man whose job was eliminated when he was age fifty-five. We had finally persevered, financially, through getting three children through college and our daughter's wedding. It was supposed to be our time to get our financial affairs in order to prepare for our future now that our kids were on their own.

"What, Your Job Was Eliminated?"

I have always said and believed that life does and can change at a moment's notice, and this was one of those moments! Suffice it to say that we went through years of marital struggle caused by this huge emotional and financial strain as we tried to reposition ourselves at this late stage of life.

There is so much to say on these tough, bleak years, but for now the purpose of this book is to convey that I understand what other Boomers have gone or are going through and how absolutely devastating it is to have the bottom fall out of what was thought to be a secure life.

Bob did eventually start working for a wonderful company, and he still is working past the "normal" retirement age. Delayed retirement is another major reason for my passion for my fellow Boomers; so many of us are forging our own way in this new Boomer frontier of aging and in the timing of it all—nothing is the same as it used to be.

Things have not worked out like millions of us Boomers thought they would.

And where is the norm? What happened to the way it used to be, with companies and pensions and thirty-plus career years?

And what about our health care needs? Will we have

the money to take care of medical issues that may or may not be covered?

And in my own interior design business I have had to reinvent myself over and over due to the Internet, HGTV, recession years, and now a very crowded interior designer field.

So what is the answer to all these "wonderful, life-changing events"?

A new MINDSET is an absolute must!

I repeat and will keep repeating that things are changing swiftly in America, and we must prepare ourselves in a totally different mindset in order to literally survive what is ahead.

Boomers must "make up their minds" to take charge of their health through smarter lifestyle choices to live the quality of life they so deserve.

Boomers must "make up their minds" to take charge of their future living spaces by acknowledging the need to upgrade their homes to live the quality of life they so deserve. And Bob and I are doing and have done just this very thing by renovating our home, Cypress, to meet our needs now and in our future. Even though we were ahead of our time to do the "aging in place" thing, and were thought to be crazy for taking on such a huge project at our age, we have reaped our rewards of pioneer thinking and doing, as we absolutely love, love, love Cypress in terms of function, safety, beauty, and restorative sanctuary spaces.

Plus, I actually cook. And, I actually cook healthy and strive for other smarter lifestyle choices. And, guess what? This is a MINDSET also. I hear over and over and over again how "it is only me" or "just the two of us" or "I am working and don't have time."

I am going to harshly say "baloney!" This is a compromised negative stronghold that will be us Boomers' demise if we do not get a hold of our daily decisions of how to live better and smarter. This is not about "look at me, I actually cook just for myself or for Bob and me," but to prove the point of IT DOESN'T MATTER IF IT IS JUST YOU OR JUST THE TWO OF YOU. The point is to develop new or better or different mindsets that will secure a better, healthier, and more secure future.

The clock is ticking, dear Boomers, and it is critical to change or get a new MINDSET on aging and preparing for the future. Boy, this is a hard message to deliver, but again, I believe my fellow Boomers who are aiming to age eloquently will not only receive this message, but adopt a new MINDSET for themselves.

Not one single person in this whole universe can do this for the Boomer. Only the Boomer can control their MIND; and where their MIND goes, that Boomer's future will certainly follow. You'll see.

Live Your Boomer Wisdom by Knowing and Doing Boomer Smarts

It is no secret that most interior designers are right-brain thinkers, which means having a creative mind versus a logical, nontechnical math kind of mind. And for sure, that is me...a right-brain creative visionary!

So, what's the big issue going on here? Why would this be part of a chapter on mindsets? Oh, my, if you only knew. Years ago, I began observing in my interior design business that my clients' homes were, for the most part, not meeting their needs on so many levels. I would get so frustrated at the "wrongness" of what is offered today in home spaces and even more frustrated when the client wanted me to "just make it all better" for them—how does one make a huge wrong a right?

I started processing how, easily, over three-fourths of

what I see in the homes of family, friends, and clients is grossly inadequate to meet their needs. And this was even before my passion developed for wanting to prepare Boomers for preparing their homes for their later years.

"Bingo!" I thought. I'll do a blog, and write and photograph on these exact issues. I'll get out there and teach and educate and inspire others to think about their homes in ways not previously considered.

"Uh, Mitzi," I then thought, "you have not the slightest idea how to do all the technical requirements to have an online blog. What is your URL, domains, and so on?" Another bingo! Only this time in the form of a mental hurdle, and another huge battle with my MINDSET against learning and doing technical skills that will only take me ten times longer than most people to learn and relearn and learn and relearn in order for any concept to actually stick in my right-brain mind, for Pete's sake.

I would get so utterly discouraged and overwhelmed that it would have been so easy to just pitch this whole idea and say, "Nice try, but this is just way too hard, and why are you possibly thinking you can pull this off, anyway? Who do you think you are at 'your age,' doing what all those younger and much smarter techie bloggers are already accomplishing...really, Mitzi...get real with yourself!"

> "For as he [or she!] thinks in his heart, so is he."
> —Proverbs 23: 7

EXACTLY!

Day in and day out, my MINDSET had to keep believing that I can do and learn whatever it is to accomplish my passion and my goal of helping my fellow Boomers do it differently and do it better on aging in America.

How did I do this? Well, first off, I am a strict believer

in knowing that whatever I do not know, there are others who certainly do. The challenge, of course, was finding those that could help me. But, eventually, they came into my life. Bob has definitely pitied them as they scratched their heads or rolled their eyes at my total incompetence!

But the big but here is the obvious. I had to simply make up my mind that in order to do what I believe I am called to do, no matter how tedious and frustrating this part of my Boomer endeavor is, my fellow Boomers are worth it! I must keep on keeping on trying, messing up, trying again, messing up—and still to this day, that is my pattern. I mess up a lot!

Big secret: WHERE THE BOOMER MIND GOES, THE BOOMER WILL CERTAINLY FOLLOW.

If we allow negative thoughts to dominate our mindsets, such as, "I am too old, I am too far gone in my health to have a chance again, I don't have the money, I don't have the skills or education," we certainly will stay stuck exactly where we are. So sad, and so unnecessary and futile when a new mindset can open up a new life potential we never dreamed could happen.

We were created to be visual beings. This means if we can see something in our minds, visualize it, we can move toward that image. Therefore, if we see ourselves as unhealthy or fat or stuck in a mundane life, plodding through our days, guess what? That mental vision is exactly what will be the reality until, and unless, a new MINDSET or a new vision is formed. Until we can see it, it simply cannot happen.

I see myself going higher and higher in my technical skills. I see myself getting healthier, not weaker and plagued with aging symptoms. I see Bob and me finishing Cypress as I visualize the projects not yet accomplished. I see my children and grandchildren successful.

Argue all you want, but this works. I am the example

of this premise of visualization and belief that I can and I will accomplish my goals—of course, not without help and not without tons of patience and tons of time and tons of effort. I am not talking magic here.

So time will tell on my own personal story, as you will witness whether I make it or not.

My MINDSET, however, tells me that what I am visualizing for my future will indeed surely follow. And I am certainly no smarter, richer, better educated, or more connected than all of my beloved Boomers. I am simply one Boomer that has made up her MIND to age differently and to age better in America. AND, to bring along with me all my fellow Boomers who have MADE UP THEIR MINDS to age differently and age better in America.

I can see (visualize) it all now. Can you?

Me, Refused?
You Have to Be Kidding!

As I wrote at the beginning of this chapter, even though I pay extra for supplemental insurance, a doctor refused to see me simply because I was insured by Medicare. No matter, I am now a Medicare person as far as the health care industry is concerned.

While this affects other Boomers, too, I needed to assess and process and most definitely change my own personal MINDSET regarding how I approach getting older. "What?" I thought at the time. "She doesn't know me or why I called or how hard I have worked to stay in great health and not be a drain on the system, and all she can tell me is 'sorry, we do not take any Medicare patients.' "

Truly, I felt like I had been kicked in the stomach! What does this mean for my future health care needs? What if something happens to the doctors whose system I am currently in? What would I do and who would accept me as a patient?

I do not hear many of my fellow Boomers talking about this bigger-than-life issue. Are they all going to be as shocked and even stunned as I was when they hear "sorry, we are not taking any more Medicare patients"?

So you know what? Right then and there, I made the choice to change my MINDSET on how I proceeded towards my future. No more just assuming that all is well and all will work out and all that other Pollyanna kind of thinking. This kind of thinking believes that because we have worked hard and are of "age," we assume and expect our government social systems to perhaps not take care of all our needs but at least to not be THE OBSTACLE in obtaining our basic needs in our health and in our future living environments.

You can do anything you decide to do. You can act to change and control your life; and the procedures the process is its own reward.

—Amelia Earhart

Now realize that I am a very positive person and a woman of deep and ever-growing faith who believes I will indeed have a beautiful future ahead regardless of my age.

But I also see reality when it smacks me right in the face! "Sorry, we are not taking any more Medicare patients."

I can see it now...a new and bulging Boomer Smart movement across America that wakes up and says, "Are you kidding me?"

This could be a Woodstock revisited protest across America, waking up and shaking up this beyond huge 78 million strong Boomer demographic to possess and activate a new MINDSET regarding hard-earned and deserved Social Security and Medicare benefits.

So what do George W. Bush, Bill Clinton, Laura Bush, Loni Anderson, Dolly Parton, Liza Minnelli, Jimmy Buffett, Donald Trump, Diane Keaton, Tommy Lee Jones, and me, yours truly, have in common? We are all part of the elite group of being amongst the oldest of Baby Boomers. Now you might ask, "So what does this have to do with Boomer Smarts begetting Boomer Power?" Well, take a look at these and others in this elite group of THE leading edge of this Boomer generation and see for yourself who has had the mindset of aging with Boomer Smarts.

We can "hide" our lifestyle pretty easily until getting into our sixties, and then we are very often like a public billboard of how or whether we have incorporated living in a Smart Boomer way or in a "whatever" mindset on our own personal aging.

Now, of course, life happens. We all acknowledge that, regardless of lifestyle, physical issues do occur. But, in general, we are what we have lived in mind, body, and spirit...period. There is just far too much evidence to prove this strong statement declaring we have a say in our futures by our MINDSETS!

Where the Boomer Mind Goes, the Boomer Will Surely Follow

These examples from the Mayo Clinic show us how an

institute as prestigious as THE Mayo Clinic views the power of positive thinking.

I've never done it before.
It's an opportunity to learn something new.

It's too complicated.
I'll tackle it from a different angle.

I don't have the resources.
Necessity is the mother of invention.

It's too radical to change.
Let's take a chance.

I'm not going to get any better at this.
I'll give it another try.

The good news in this wonderfully empowering fact: it is never too late to change our MINDSETS about aging and begin again. We are so amazingly resilient in mind, body, and spirit that anything is possible if we change our minds regarding how we will age.

Boomers must come to grips with this fact of life: we are indeed aging. But we are and will do it differently, being more active and more engaged socially, financially, and spiritually than previous generations because, after all, we are the Baby Boomers who never do anything like everyone else.

Knowing Without Doing Is Not Living a Boomer Smart Life

Researchers continue to explore the effects of positive thinking and optimism on health, and this is exactly what having a Boomer Smart MINDSET is all about!

Mayo Clinic:

Health benefits of a HEALTHY MINDSET:
- Increased life span.
- Lower rates of depression.
- Greater resistance to the common cold.
- Lower levels of distress.
- Better psychological and physical well-being.
- Reduced risk of death from cardiovascular disease.
- Better coping skills during hardships and times of stress.

DECLARING AND DESIGNING YOUR BEST BOOMER LIFE all starts in the mind...making up our minds that we will indeed and without a doubt have a fabulous future.
How?
By believing with a new MINDSET that we can be healthy as we age by learning and embracing new lifestyles that daily restore our energy and raise our quality of life by intentional and functional planning for our futures.
By believing with a new MINDSET that we can live in homes that daily restore our energy and quality of life by intentional and functional planning of our lives.
Our mind is our mental house. Our life will follow our thoughts or MINDSETS.
Therefore, you need to remodel your mental house.

In Your Health

DECLARE your health is getting stronger and better daily.

Mindsets

DECLARE you eat to live your very best life for yourself and in order to be your best for those you care so much about.

DECLARE you daily live in peace and joy as you control the stresses of your life.

DECLARE you exercise and are experiencing renewed energy and releasing stresses.

DECLARE your new lifestyle of getting eight hours of sleep and practicing a balanced life to live your best life now and in your future.
In Your Home

DECLARE you have a personal restorative sanctuary space in your home.

DECLARE your present or future home will take you into your future years with style, dignity, and a fabulous quality of life.

DECLARE your present or future home will give you so much joy that it renews and restores your energy daily.

DECLARE your present or future home provides all your physical needs now and in your future.

Now, Being Equipped, Enlightened, and Empowered with Boomer Smart Mindsets, You Are Declaring and Designing Your Best Boomer Life Now!

You'll See.

Questions for Chapter 2: Mindsets

1. If you could let yourself dream big for doing or becoming something, what would it be?

2. How long has your mind been entertaining the "what ifs" for this dream or goal?

3. What would it take for you to seriously consider your first steps in making your dream or goal a reality?

4. If you could be truly honest with yourself, beside the normal money and time restraints and age and all the normal excuses, what really is holding you back from pursuing your dreams or goals?

Mindsets

Boomer Smart Stories

Leslie Carothers
Messages of Hope
www.MessagesOfHope.com
www.TKPartnership.com

the kaleidoscope partnership

Mitzi: It's been exciting doing these interviews. I am just thrilled with the response and the forthrightness of women to share to help other women. It's been really cool.

Well, anyway, so you and I were talking on Mindsets, and this is how women, men, too, but mainly we're dealing with women when they reach a certain age, many have the mindset that, "It's over. It's done. How can I possibly do this? I'm too old. I don't have the money. I don't have the contacts."

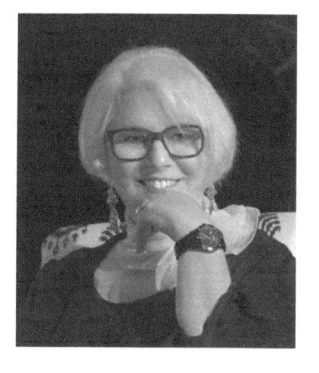

It's mindset. And mindset, as we know, Leslie, can be positive, negative, but it's never benign. It will move us in one direction or another.

And so, the question, the first question I have for you, is what significant life event altered your future plans that you have anticipated would be your designated, or your calculated, or what you thought your future was going to look like? What was that event?

Leslie: The death of my father by pancreatic cancer.

Mitzi: Where were you living?

Leslie: I was actually living in Houston when we first

found out that my father had cancer. And then when he passed away, I moved back to Florida, which is where my mother was living and had been living—and they'd been married for fifty-one years. And so, there she was, and it was very sudden. My dad actually contracted cancer and he was dead five weeks later. So the progression of the disease was extremely fast, and no one had been...he was seemingly healthy and then he was dead in five weeks. So, you know, none of us had had time to prepare for that in any way, and least of all my mom. And just seeing that, you know, she really needed—I mean, I needed support as well and so did she, and I was free to move to Florida. So, I did.

Mitzi: You were north in Minneapolis.

Leslie: Well, I was, and so, after living in Florida for a couple of years and going through a lot of personal, professional turmoil there for two years, I actually took a job assignment up in Minneapolis that I thought was going to be for three months and turned into three years. And that moving to Minneapolis became, I would say, the full circle upon which my life completely changed into something, if you will.

So, it was really the events following the death of my dad by pancreatic cancer that led me then to Minneapolis that absolutely did change the course of my life in the second half.

Mitzi: And how did you respond to this life-changing reset, talking about going to Minneapolis, picking it up from there? You left Florida. You went to Minneapolis, and what was your...what was your new direction? I mean, what did you think your life was going to be like in Minneapolis and did it happen?

Leslie: I actually really had no idea. Well, yes, I did have an idea when I went there because I went for a work assignment that I thought was actually going to turn into something different than what it turned into. And when it didn't turn into what I thought it was going to turn into, I was really completely directionless. And it was at that time that I had this powerful dream for Messages of Hope, to actually buy the domain name. So it truly was—yes, it truly was during that time of trying to find my way again that I actually did have the dream to buy the domain name, which made me get up in the middle of the night to buy it.

Mitzi: And—well, then you—when you found yourself in an unknown situation, so to speak, and—

Leslie: Completely. [Laughs]

Mitzi: It was—well, I love your word directionless, that—did it shake your booties? I mean did you freak out or were you somewhere in between when your plans didn't work out? How did you "re-center" yourself?

Leslie: To answer your specific question, what I decided to do when I found myself directionless in Minneapolis for a bit was to get healthy, really, and I spent a year of my life there—my first year there, really. After things didn't work out exactly the way I had intended, I actually made it my job to get healthy and I lost 50 pounds. I went to Weight Watchers. Yup, I exercised—

Mitzi: I love that, Leslie. So, you did not—I'm not paraphrasing or putting words but observing what you're saying—you weren't wallowing in self-pity without—

Leslie: No.

Mitzi: ...taking some action, and moving forward is what you've been doing.

Leslie: Absolutely. Absolutely not. I just went on. "I'm not made that way." I made that way for about two days or three days or maybe a week but—[Laughs]

Mitzi: Exactly. So, you—

Leslie: I think we all need to wallow a little bit. [Laughs]

Mitzi: Yes. Oh, my goodness, yes. We—that's kind of grieving, you know, when you'd had a loss of—you will grieve a loss of the job. It may not be the same as a parent, of course, we both lost our fathers and we must of course grieve at a different level, but still we have acknowledged what's going on in our lives. Otherwise, I see people all the time that are just bearing it all under "I am fine, thank you." Then, it comes out in not-so-cool ways, you know, anger and sarcasm and all that kind of stuff. So were those good years?

Leslie: They were excellent years, yes. One of my biggest—when my first really big social media client came because of living there, and that was Cargill. Cargill is the largest, you know, privately held company in the U.S., and they had a division of theirs named BiOH Polyols; they actually hired me to run their entire social media campaign and they're headquartered in Minneapolis.
So, living in Minneapolis, and they wanted to work with someone local. So, living there directly led to complete immersion of my business.

Mindsets

Mitzi: Oh, wow. Everybody that I know of loves Minneapolis.

Leslie: I agree. I loved it, too, you know.

Mitzi: So now, then, what led you away from this fine situation?

Leslie: Yeah, it was a great situation there, but really what led me away from it I would say was my time on Twitter and really recognizing how many—this is really true, recognizing I did not have to move back to Houston. I mean there was no financial need for me to move back to Houston. There was no—there was absolutely nothing pushing me to move back to Houston.

The only thing that really happened that moved me back to Houston was really my time on social media. I'm seeing, and not because of conversations I personally was having, but just seeing through my Twitter stream how many people were actually losing their parents. This is really exactly what happened, and I saw how sad they were, and, of course, I had gone through that, my dad, and I thought, I only have my mom left.

So I was living in Minneapolis. My brother was living here in Houston, and so, I was two years into living in Minneapolis and that year, that second year, I went back to Florida for the summer. We packed, and my mom, she sold her home, and my brother had several homes here. And so, my brother and sister-in-law, they moved her into one of their homes five minutes from where they live here.

So, all of a sudden I don't have a brother in Houston and a mother in Florida. I have a brother in Houston where I had already lived for twenty years of my life, living within five minutes of my mother.

And I'm up in Minneapolis. So, there was no one. I mean, I had lived in Houston twenty years prior to moving back to Florida for those two years after my dad died of cancer. So, Houston was really my adult home for twenty years. And I also started thinking—you know, I don't have children, so for me to stay up in Minneapolis, even, until my seventies and eighties where temperatures often are negative zero. That doesn't make sense. You don't have to live there when you're old. It's probably not where you want to live when you're old. I love it there, except for when I was in my fifties, but I didn't see loving it in later years. I thought, you know, if I stay here for the rest of my life, which I could have, I—not having children or family there, it's not easy to get around when you're elderly in Minneapolis.

So, I was really just looking ahead and saying there's not a reason for me to stay there. My brother and mother live five minutes from each other, and I lived here for twenty years. And so, now it's time for me to come back. And so I did. I made the decision to come back.

Mitzi: That is what we're trying to encourage, for other Boomers to look at their future and evaluate if where they are is where they want to be in the future, and that's exactly what you did. What are you doing? The next and last question is what are you doing, for I know the answer to this, I think, but what are you doing presently that will prepare your future years to be purposeful and productive?

Leslie: Yes, I have actually started. I am building and we're going to launch at the end of this year a website called MessagesOfHope.com. And the purpose of Messages of Hope is to support the charities that the site's buyers believe in.

So, we're turning the charity model on its head, as you will. Normally when you go to a website, a certain percentage these days of whatever your purchase is will go to some charity or another that the websites' owners care about or have made the beneficiary of their work. And I'm actually turning that model upside down, and the site's buyers will actually be able to choose the charity they care about to support with their purchases.

And the—that has not ever been done before, and was the direction that I was really given by God, the universe, to go in, like the site, which was to make it a place where other people could choose which charity they want to support, what is meaningful to them versus me choosing to donate a portion of the proceeds of the site's purchases to a charity that I care about. And then because I don't have children, as soon as I'm able to, I will turn the charity into a non-profit.

Mitzi: Beautiful.

Leslie: ...in addition, I will up the amount that I'm able to donate, or that the non-profit donates to the charities. And so—

Mitzi: Wow.

Leslie: ...in that way...in that way, in mind—I hope that would be a legacy of what's really important to me.

Mitzi: Yes. It's beautiful. It really is. And that's part of what is so purposeful and meaningful, to leave a legacy, have that influence while we are here, and then to leave a legacy when we're gone. And that certainly is there in Messages of Hope. It's a real model and inspiration and it's something tangible.

Leslie: ...yup. And so, the site will have both. The domain name, which is what came to me in this very powerful dream, is, I think, what will power the sales of the site, although I don't know that yet. But the keyword "hope" on Google has sixteen and a half million hits a month. So, the whole site, every part that's on the site, is optimized around the keyword hope, and everything, every e-card, every profit on the site, is something that speaks to hope. So if you saw something on the site, you're going to think I have a friend that's in the hospital or a nursing home or sick or just broke up with somebody or, you know, whatever—someone may be having a hard time—you might want to send them a little gift of hope. And you'll be able to do it on this site and find it on this site, and you'll be able to find e-cards, which you can send for, I don't know, whatever it's going to be, a dollar or two dollars. And you can fill them with messages of hope and they'll fly over to them.

I mean, a product of some sort that you design that relates to hope, it would need to be exclusive, and some people are doing jewelry. Robin's a jewelry artist who is doing little art pieces. And she's also doing e-cards. I mean, there are probably right now about twenty people doing different things right now.

Mitzi: Excellent. It's so exciting. So—

Leslie: It's really exciting. I'm so excited. [Laughs]

Mitzi: Yes, and people—everybody—well, not everybody,

but most of us want to be involved in something that is outside of ourselves for the good of others. And it's just such a win-win because, you know, the adage "we all receive more than we give" is exactly what this is, and so—

Leslie: It really is.

Mitzi: And you know, I can hear the joy in your voice when you talk about it, love when you—

Leslie: Oh.

Mitzi: …that's exactly why I mean you are so blessed, Leslie; the prospect of how much this is going to help others to still hope by somebody caring about them. It's just a beautiful, beautiful thing, Leslie.

Leslie: Thank you.

Mitzi: You're so welcome. So, the last question, then. What advice would you give your fellow Boomers at their crossroads when their pre-determined plan experienced a train wreck or they must change directions for various reasons? You are a survivor, so to speak. How did you get there? What advice would you tell other Boomers when they're in their fifties or even their sixties and they think, "Oh, my goodness, nothing is working here. What am I going to do?" I know it's a difficult question, but you took a year off to take care of yourself, and I think the wisdom in that rather than scrambling and just trying to try this or try that, is that part of your advice?

Leslie: I do absolutely. I would say the first thing for me

is truly my faith that ever directs every step that I take. Every step we take is being directed by the universe. So I would say just the word faith. I would just say we really have faith, and really, Mitzi, I have had very unusual dreams—a lot of my life since I was thirty years old. I know one hundred percent that this is not the only level that we actually exist on. It's really true.

I would just say, and however people are experiencing that, whether they believe in the Heaven and Earth model or some other model of faith. That's if it is someone else's perspective that because you are fifty or older and this is just not possible…well, none of this is true.

And usually these things relate to money, you know, really at the end of the day. Or usually a lot of things like that—or catastrophes we see as Boomers just relate to some loss of income or health.

Mitzi: Exactly.

Leslie: You know, one of the two.

Mitzi: That's right.

Leslie: It's one of those two things. And so, the loss of income thing, there are so many resources and I would really say to our Boomer, get on social media. Get on LinkedIn. Understand that—and I'll just give you a personal experience.

My mother at seventy-four, who never touched a computer in her life and thought she would never ever do it, when my dad died, she actually took herself off to the community college and sat down, she did. And now, she's eighty-three and she sits for hours a day and plays bridge, which is her hobby online, with people from all over the world.

Mitzi: Cool.

Leslie: It's true. My mother even buys things online. Let me tell you seriously, my mother, up and down, she would never touch a computer. Right after my dad died and I suggested it to her, absolutely not, not ever, and she finally came to that place where she realized she'd be incredibly out of it and probably incredibly lonely, and so she did. She went to a community college and then she asked for my brother and I to help her once in a while, and she's learned all on her own, nobody teaching her. So, I would say to other Boomers, it's never too late to learn the computer.

And I believe that as you get older, being familiar even on Twitter can be invaluable. On Sunday mornings I participate in something called the Spirit Chat, and there's a woman that's on that chat that's in her eighties and her name on Twitter is Grandma on Deck. Her real name is Gloria and she keeps herself really active through communicating with other people. So, I would, again, I would say—yes. So, I think, really truly, especially for older people, I believe that communicating via social media allows you to have a life and to use your mind. So, if your body can't move even if you're straight out in bed and you're sick, you have cancer or something that's horrible, right?

Mitzi: Right.

Leslie: If you can type, you can be connected to the world.

Mitzi: And I think you and I agree that there is a destiny for all of us. And if we can allow that to come forth, then we live that out. And instead of fighting what is not meant to be, there are different opportunities at different life stages. It doesn't mean that we stay in the same place in all stages. I think that's where we find that so many Boomers run into trouble. But it's just when our plan doesn't work out, then many will freak. And stories like yours are about 'let it go.' There's another better plan, normally. So—

Leslie: I actually really think there always is. I think what you have to really do is to go—to get quiet inside your heart. I think you really sometimes have to give up or at least be willing—not have to but to be willing to give up all the material stuff and just say, "Okay, if I didn't have this house or this car or this, all of these, if I didn't have to—if I didn't have it and I truly was free to do any…" I mean this question is so obvious but it really—and if I go back to my childhood and remember what gave me joy, a lot of times we get stuck in what we think we have to do because of the perceptions of our family or friends or colleagues. Or like, even what your kids will think. But at the end of the day, especially for the Boomer, if you have children, what they wanted to see in their parents is just to be happy. And you can't live for your kids anyway. You know, they're not going to live for you. So at the end of the day, it's great to have financial security, so that you do feel a cushion of that underneath you. But even if you don't have that, you can still be just completely happy in the moment because you really don't know what that moment holds [Laughs].

Mitzi: Good point. Leslie, that is wonderful because this book is about hope, which of course so relates to your Messages of Hope endeavor. Everything we're talking about from the spaces all the way through the spiritual,

Mindsets

and the in between chapters on Boomer mindset, attitude, lifestyle, togetherness, is to position Boomers to hope in expectation for their future. The whole book is geared to our future preparation. So tons of us Boomers thank you for sharing all your insight and your "HOPE."

Lynne Barton Bier
Home on the Range Interiors
www.HomeOnTheRangeInteriors.com

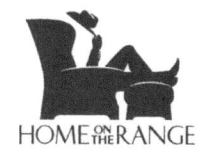

Mitzi: What life-changing event has brought you to the place where you find yourself now?

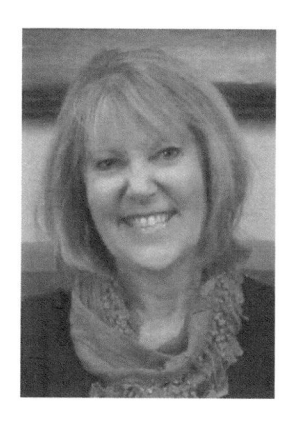

Lynne: It was really a combination of two events. My husband was fighting chronic fatigue and fibromyalgia for years, and no one seemed to be able to diagnose it as he got sicker and sicker. It turns out he had celiac disease that entire time and, by eating wheat, was poisoning himself every day. The road to recovery was a long one because his body and immune system had been weakened so much. Right about the time he was being diagnosed, 9-11 happened, and then the tech crash. We had a large ski-in, ski-out property that we had been renting out that became vacant, and since it was quite large and in a prime location, no one wanted to take the risk of starting a new business in it in a tough economy. I knew that I had already started, grown, and sold two home furnishing and interior design businesses (sold to focus on design and my children for six years), and I knew I could do it again, so I started another home furnishing store in my late forties and ran it along with my interior design business.

Mitzi: What prompted this effort of social media and working with your daughter Payje plus your new business scopes? How did you make it happen?

Lynne: I have always been intimately involved in all aspects of my business and am always on the search for new ways to market it and ways to adapt to changes in the market and technology. I was the first design and home furnishing business in Steamboat to create a website and shared the cost of having a professional photographer shoot the houses I was working on with the architect and builders.

As time went on, I realized that we needed to keep adapting so that our website wouldn't get stagnant. About that time, I went to a presentation by *Mountain Living Magazine* on Digital Sherpa and then Design Sherpa, and I hired them to create a blog for us. At the same time, my daughter Payje was learning how to set up her own websites and created a blog on couponing and photography that later turned into a wonderful travel blog. I realized I wasn't getting any younger, and that I needed to do some things that were "out of the box" for me to stimulate my creativity.

I decided that attending the Design Blogger's Convention in LA would give me the impetus I needed to really delve into the world of social media. That was a turning point for me and helped launch me into Houzz, Pinterest, Facebook, Twitter, and Olioboard. When Payje decided to move back to Steamboat with her boyfriend, I realized that I felt like a drowning person who was being rescued from the depths. Keeping up with all of the social media platforms, learning all of the tools necessary, and spending the time necessary to keep it all going—at the same time I was running a design business and retail store—was total insanity. My average workweek was eighty hours, and my quality of life was at an all-time low. Involving Payje allowed me to turn over the social media and marketing side of the business to someone who had the creativity, technical know-how, and excellent writing skills needed to make that part of the business flourish. I was able to go back to focusing on the design and retail portion of the business and keep it growing.

Mitzi: What does your life look like now versus your "before life"?

Lynne: I have been able to build another very successful design business, create homes for people that give them a vacation getaway from their own hectic lives, and have time for travel and for my "children."
   I still work harder than I would ideally like, but I have realized that a good part of that is my personality, and that if I weren't working, I would be volunteering just as much. I have become more accepting of who I am, and have realized that what is important to me is surrounding myself with people who enjoy their lives as well. I love building friendships with my clients and maintaining those friendships over the years. I find time to travel with my friends and my children and have been checking destinations off my "bucket list."

Mitzi: What advice would you give to other Boomers when their lives go off course from what they had planned for their Boomer years?

Lynne: Always look for ways to turn adversity into something positive.

Rather than sitting around bemoaning what has happened to your life, look for ways to change it around.

Stimulate your mind with new experiences and opportunities to learn new things. Start every day thinking of something you are grateful for.

Make time for your friends and family.

Do something you are passionate about as often as possible—for me it is travel.

Create quiet alone time when you can read, take walks, contemplate the universe, or whatever relaxes you.

Give yourself credit for your successes—I always have a hard time with this one!!

Of course the proverbial eat well and exercise because your mental and emotional being works better when you take care of your body.

Mitzi: Well, you should be writing your own book with all these words of wisdom, Lynne! Awesome, a simply and perfectly awesome ending, and you have contributed immensely to Boomers everywhere. Thank you.

Chapter 3
Attitudes

Ageless Aging with a Boomer Smart Attitude

Paradigm: example, pattern, model, standard, criterion, prototype

Shortsighted: lacking foresight, ill-considered, unwise, ill-advised, unthinking, heedless, rash

Strong-willed: determined, resolute, stubborn, obstinate, headstrong, self-willed, inflexible, intractable

Attitudes in Our Boomer Homes

I was recently having a conversation with a couple of my older Boomer clients; they were in their early sixties and asked if I could review their new house plans to see if there were areas to upgrade for their "future years."

Without a second's hesitation, their response to my ideas was, "Oh, we'll do those things later." And in such a firm, non-compromising tone of voice that I knew this conversation was forever closed to them and, furthermore, I was not to bring this up again!

Yikes...okay, okay, already. Paradigms? Shortsighted? Strong-willed?

What does "we will do those things later" really mean?

I think it actually means, "Don't bug me, Mitzi. I will never fall, have surgery or knee or hip replacement, or have an accident that prevents me from using my bathroom. Come on, I don't want to hear about this, let alone consider doing the changes or upgrades that you are talking about. Don't bug me with this upgrade for this future use stuff!"

Attitudes on Our Boomer Health

Bob and I were at dinner with friends our age and the conversation came up about what meds we were on, as if this is normal dinner conversation. We said none, really, and they couldn't believe we were not at least on high blood pressure medicine or a statin to control our cholesterol or any arthritis meds. Their comments were, "Well, every one of our friends is taking at least some of these, just like us."

Sadly, this is the herd mentality. "Everyone else is like us, so what's the big deal here?"

Paradigms? Shortsighted? Strong-willed?

What was really being expressed here? I think our friends' comments expose the American way for many Boomers, which is you get older, you have an issue, you go to the doctor and get meds for it. Period, end of story. Don't talk to me about changing my ways. I am just like everyone else!

In the planning of an extensive and very expensive kitchen remodel, I asked the client how they would use their kitchen, meaning how did they work their daily cooking? The answer was, "Oh, for delivery or take-in foods and maybe just cook lunch or breakfast here. We go out to eat almost every night."

What was really being said here, and what was the attitude? It was probably, "Are you kidding me? Cook with

Attitudes

our crazy schedule?" Or, "It is just me or just me and my spouse, so why would I go to all that trouble? Seriously, Mitzi, that is so not the way we are going to live in this stage."

Paradigms? Stubborn? Strong-willed?

Seriously, this is way common, no matter the economic level, as we all so well know the fast food statistics and eating out as the main food source for the American diet. BUT this is not true for those with Boomer Smart Attitudes...no way are these Boomers getting sucked into that self-defeating pattern of thinking.

Enter the Boomer with Boomer Smart Attitudes, and this is what is heard:

In Home

While looking at a possible new home purchase with clients to evaluate the appropriateness of the home's layout, the wife said, "I know we will have to remodel this master bathroom. Look how narrow this door is, and check out this way-outdated and unsafe shower. We may not do it right away, but we know we have to do this upgrade." This wise client grasped the concepts and realities of accident free and ease of living principles that will benefit her every day for years to come. Boomer Smart Attitude, for sure.

In Health

A friend was telling me about how his doctor prescribed a statin drug for high cholesterol, which he did not fill in order to try diet and exercise first to see if the drug was necessary. After he changed his diet and eating routines, at the next checkup the doctor says, "Great job, your cholesterol is down from 200 to 185. The statins are working." My friend never filled that prescription but took the bull by the horns and said, "I am going to be proactive on my health and not start this long road of one med after another." Boomer Smart Attitude, for sure.

I was once doing a TV taping on Boomer Smart Cooking, showing how easy it was to prepare a simple, healthy, yummy, and fast meal, and the comments I kept hearing were, "This is so easy if I just plan my meals instead of waiting till I am exhausted at the end of the day and give in and stop and pick something up that I know is not good for me." Definitely more Boomer Smart Attitudes coming alive, for sure.

AGELESS Aging with a Boomer Smart Attitude is the key, in my opinion, to a great life ahead for all of us Boomers—no matter where we are coming from in our health and in our homes. This has absolutely nothing to do with our present or past circumstances, but how we CHOOSE our attitudes towards those present or past circumstan-ces that will make or break achieving Boomer Smarts in all areas.

Attitudes Affect Aging!

This is what I call the Triple A's of Aging. I have spoken on this for years, watching those in a class or audience, waiting for the light bulbs to go on for the ones that get it, and inside I am cheering a big yes for them!

But have you ever watched someone silently but visibly, with their facial expressions or body language, tell you that, "Lady, you are smoking bananas here and I am not buying one word of what you are telling us"?

Well I certainly have because what we are believing, teaching, and writing says that aging is all about our own attitudes, and sorry to say, many of our Boomers adamantly do not want to hear this because—here

Attitudes

goes—it wipes out all their excuses.

Okay, I am really ducking here, but I have always been out there in my thinking, believing, and doing. Why else, for heaven's sake, would I even be doing this whole Boomer aging thing in the first place?

Because I care deeply about my fellow Boomers. If this effort helps even some to open their eyes and ears to what is happening in America, motivating them to what they need to do to prepare for these changes, then it all is definitely worth it.

Real change always begins in our minds. This is why we must examine our attitudes and not our circumstances.

It is time for us Boomers to shake off that stinking thinking old age mentality. It is time for us to choose to rise above the stereotype of aging in America and become the "new normal" of aging with style, dignity, class, and, most importantly, influence.

So how are you preparing for your future? Are you even thinking about your future let alone preparing for it?

Well, if your answer is simply a no, you are not alone. Unfortunately, that is my huge concern for my fellow Boomers and America because in just a few short years, what we have come to expect of our government may not be the new reality of Social Security or Medicare, which have been historically relied on by millions of Americans.

Okay…enough already of doom and gloom statistics and predictions!

We are the Boomers…remember? THE BOOMERS! We changed America even as we were born! Remember war babies? Remember Woodstock? And rock and roll that made "the establishment" shudder?

The adage that our strengths can also be our weakness is sadly true, however. We believe we Boomers will never age, and if we do, it will be on our terms. Nice philosophy, but so sorry, this is not reality—even for us infallible Boomers.

But now we know our Boomer future holds great promise for all of us regardless of our money, status, or health.

It is all about AGING WITH A BOOMER SMART ATTITUDE.

Change your attitude, dear Boomer, and change your life. You'll see.

Garbage In, Garbage Out

I really hate to admit this, and I really might get backlash from revealing this, but I am going to do it anyway.

A while back, I was at a gathering of some very accomplished and professional interior designers. Don't even ask me why, but I stuck my silly neck out to bring up social media skills as being very critical to our business futures, and I was shocked and dismayed at what I heard.

"Well, you won't catch me putting my personal information on Facebook!"

"Well, I've heard that it's even personally dangerous!"

"Social media is so silly and childish; like who cares if I am having coffee at Starbucks?"

"Why would I ever do that now at my age?" (Meaning: "I am doing quite fine just the way I have always done my business, thank you very much.")

And the shaking of heads of those seated around the table as they agreed with these statements made me sadly realize how close-minded Boomer attitudes can be to change, to new ideas, to learning new things. They can be so unteachable from either being misinformed or pridefully arrogant, often stating, "I am doing just fine so don't mess with me." Well, alrighty then!

And it is amazingly sad to me that those conversations thwarted any discovery of the amazing potential

Attitudes

and scope of social media—like blogs and professional connections on LinkedIn or Twitter—to reach other professionals and trade and vendor opportunities. No, it is so not about "I am having coffee at Starbucks." Please!

I am sure everyone has heard the phrase garbage in/garbage out in regards to what goes in our minds, computers, bodies, and so forth. In other words, what we allow into any of these areas is exactly what comes back out.

What does any of this have to do with Boomer Smart Attitudes? Well, if we listen without a discerning ear to what is being said around us, it is very, very easy to just go with the flow of what everyone else is thinking or doing. It is also very, very easy to eat the garbage by agreeing to what others are saying just because they are our friends, family, associates, or even colleagues.

10 Attitudes That Keep Us Stuck in the Mire of Garbage Thinking

1. I'm getting old and I just can't change who I am or what I do, for heaven's sake!
2. I don't have time to exercise. I'm too busy already.
3. I don't have the time or money to work on a thing in my house.
4. This is the way I've always done things, and I don't need any help or anyone telling me how to live my life.
5. My time is valuable, and I'd like to be with my family and friends and do what I want to do. Why would I consider helping a food bank or neighborhood school? Let all those do-gooders get out there and do their thing.
6. All my friends look like I do.
7. Starting a home remodeling project is just unreal-

istic. Where would the money come from, and why would I even consider changing the way things are now?
8. Everyone I know around my age is on blood pressure medicine and a statin drug. You are crazy telling me I can get off these drugs with a change in my lifestyle.
9. When I am older, I will think about what to do with my bathroom. I certainly do not need to be upgrading for safety now.
10. Well, if I need financial help when I am older for my health or a place to live, my Medicare and Social Security benefits will take care of me.

But, of course, all ten of these stinking-garbage-type patterns of thinking keep a Boomer stuck.

Boomers *aging with an attitude*, however, are empowered, equipped, and are enlightened with *wisdom* and *understanding*.

Boomers with attitude ask:

What does my future look like?

What changes should I be making now to be healthier in my future?

Where will I live? Can I stay in my current home conveniently and safely?

Do I ever think about leaving a legacy of influence to others that lives to give?

This is one of the most critical components of a Boomer with Boomer Smart Attitudes. They know that they should not eat the garbage swirling around them everywhere, and they know they don't have to agree with everyone in "their herd" just because they all think, look, speak, or act in agreement.

Heavens, no! Boomers have always been rebels, so why are so many just going along with any ol' theory on aging

Attitudes

or any ol' housing set-ups or any ol' lifestyles in general?

The very simple explanation, indeed, is they are in need of an attitude change for sure, without a doubt, no debate, to take back their Boomer zest and return to their rebel-with-a-cause status.

My fellow Boomers who are the movers and the shakers in ageless aging are fighting hard to not give in and just look like all their friends who have just, you guessed it, given in to aging like everyone else.

But apathy and indifference are contagious. Do not hang out with these people or you can easily have their garbage thrown at you in very insidious and unsuspecting ways. Don't hang out with those people who are stuck thinking, looking, speaking, or acting in ways that go against all Boomer Smart Attitudes on ageless aging.

I know, I know—some people are just in our lives no matter what, but we do not have to seek them out over and above what is absolutely necessary, like a boss or family member. Been there, done that, too, but it doesn't mean we give lip service to agreeing or, heaven forbid, do what the Boomer slackers are doing just to go along with the herd. This is tough talking, but so is a diagnosis of diabetes due to being thirty pounds or more overweight or eating like everyone else or taking high blood pressure medicine, or falling in a grossly inadequate bathroom requiring many surgeries and physical therapy.

So who do you want to be around?

Who do you want to be like?

The really cool thing is we get to choose!

No one or nothing can chose our attitudes. No sir. It is up to each of us whether we choose to further our life with Boomer Smart Attitudes.

Thousands are already choosing a new perspective for their futures. Come join us! You will love where we are going and how we will be living. You'll see.

Boomers Get to Choose

Did you know that you can hear and discern others' levels of maturity? Yes, it is true. What are these markers of speaking that reveal a person's level of maturity and wisdom? Their words...listen to their words.

Low-Level Thinkers—Talk about other people and themselves a lot.

Mid-Level Thinkers—Talk about events and themselves a lot.

High-Level Thinkers—Talk about theories and analysis of what is happening, and concepts and philosophies or beliefs.

All of us fall in all three categories some of the time, but where we are speaking the majority of the time determines our level of maturity and wisdom. With this in mind, who do we want to hang out with? Well, for sure, Boomers equipped with Boomer Smarts know to avoid those that are:

indifferent
negative
complacent
grouchy
unteachable
uncaring
stagnant

And seek out other Boomers who are:

motivated

Attitudes

positive
compassionate
pleasant
teachable
caring
growing

Did you ever think about what you are thinking about? Did you know that you actually can choose what to think about? Most definitely, our thoughts can be controlled.

For example, someone pulls out in front of me while I am driving. I can actually choose my attitude or my thinking on how I will react. Will I shake it off and be grateful that I am not hurt, or will I become very angry thinking all sorts of non-printable adjectives toward that driver? It most certainly is my choice to choose how I will think in that very split second.

Bob had a very restless night recently, getting up many times and waking me up. After about 4:30 am, I knew getting back to sleep was not happening. I got up at 5:30, which is not uncommon when I have had a good night's sleep, but getting up at 5:30 on a poor night's sleep can set me up to think not-so-good thoughts mostly aimed right at Bob.

But I have learned the power of choice in my thoughts. Determined to not let my lack of sleep ruin my day (or Bob's), I did a lot of self-talk. "This will be a great day, Mitzi. You will get your writing done today as planned. You can take a twenty-minute nap later."

I have found controlling my thoughts to be one of my life's biggest challenges because my thoughts become my words and my words become my behaviors. Watch what words you are saying and see if this isn't the reality of how you act.

Choosing what I choose to think about is critical to my

well-being, my health, my relationships, my business, and all of my entire life. My thoughts determine my attitudes on every single thing in my life now and in my life for my future.

And again and again research, such as the huge Women's Health Initiative at the Pittsburg School of Medicine with over 100,000 women, tells us that a positive attitude affects our health. Those with a positive attitude were less likely to have heart disease because there is a definite mind-body connection.

Just tell yourself in your self-talk or your thoughts that you don't feel well and watch how your day turns out. Now we all have days where we are not up to par or fight the common cold. But I am a firm believer that how I respond to what my physical state is reflecting will without a doubt determine whether I go down for the count or simply give myself permission to have a "restore Mitzi" day. That's a totally different mindset and attitude!

This, for me, is one tough daily battle. Every day is a new day with a new set of situations to be "thought about." Some days I win my mental-thinking battles and some days I lose big time. I hate those days when I give in to self-pity, discouragement, frustration, and insecurity. But after all these years, I am very quick about thinking what I am thinking about.

Dr. Audrey Chun of the Martha Stewart Center for Living at Mount Sinai Hospital says, "One of the factors in determining aging successfully is a resilient personality/ability to recover from adversity and move on with life rather than dwell on challenges."

Dwell: to linger over in thought or speech.
—Webster's Dictionary

We cannot hear enough how our *attitudes affect* our *ag-*

ing. Yes, of course I do not keep at it all evening like I used to do. Of course I need to monitor what I eat or do not eat, discipline myself to get out there and take that walk, or the consequences are far greater than when I was in my forties. I am in my late sixties now. What I choose to dwell on regarding even my daily routine has long and far-reaching effects on this aging Boomer body, and on my mindset and attitudes.

What I choose to dwell on will determine my day, my health, my relationships, and most definitely what my future will become. It has absolutely nothing to do with actual circumstances but how I dwell or process these aging circumstances that we all have and we all evaluate one way or another.

Do we give in to it all or fight like hell? Smart Boomers are fighting like hell and will most definitely not lose this battle.

To many of my fellow Boomers, this line of "thinking" will seem irrelevant, but to those going ahead of the pack with their Boomer Smart Attitudes, I can hear the *a-has!* now.

If you listen very carefully, you will hear it and recognize this sound. It is called wisdom. Boomers with wisdom are not complainers, are not self-absorbed, but are those that are exciting and inspiring to be around.

Boomers with wisdom enjoy their life dwelling or thinking positively about what each day can bring in opportunities, whether done alone or with others.

I love Robin Williams' motto in the movie *Dead Poets Society*: carpe diem. Seize the day.

Yes, this is it exactly. We Boomers with Boomer Smarts are seizing our days to move us higher and higher in achieving our Boomer Power living.

Choose to think about what you are thinking about your future. Your life will surely change. You'll see.

Boomer Smart Stories

Cynthia Bogart
The Daily Basics
www.TheDailyBasics.com

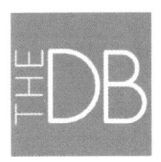

Mitzi: I've been talking to women all over the country, and you're all women of influence. And this is just really a fun-filled way to connect through social media.

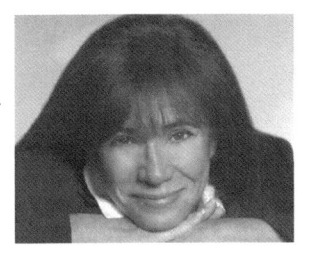

Cynthia: It's—well, it's really exciting, and you know, the whole Internet has brought us all together, and there are so many great things happening out there. So, this is exciting that you're doing this, what a great project.

Mitzi: Thank you. It has been just a passion, and actually an observation for years, that just recently in the last years how quickly and drastically things are changing in America and how this is going to have such a profound effect on Baby Boomers. And those Boomers are, as I've said, 78 million, and anyone born from 1946 through 1964. So, the oldest is 67 and the youngest is 50. And this is the wealthiest and often most highly educated group; a very effective, powerful group. But yet what I'm observing in lots of the Boomer women, especially, is the lack of awareness on what actually could and should be considered to prepare all these Boomers for what's next in all these changes. So,

Attitudes

therein lies the purpose of the book.

Cynthia: Great.

Mitzi: You know, it's just—it's so easy, isn't it, Cynthia, to get caught up in our day-to-day busyness. We're all there. And to think about our own health and our homes, will they look out for us? Do we want to stay here? Is this my last best place? I mean all of those things.

As a designer, I'm privy to a lot of upfront and personal information about my clients; for example, when I'm designing a kitchen, I know how they eat. I know because they tell me. I have to know that to know how to design their kitchen. Are they carryout? Are they fast food? Are they gourmet cooks? Do they entertain?

So, I've gained a ton of information over the years on that, and then on homes. I can tell you there are clients that I have that are in their fifties and early sixties and high-end residential, and I won't talk about aging in place, I'll just suggest doing whatever. We don't say raised toilet seats, we say comfort-height toilet—just ergonomic kitchen pullouts and things like this. And yet, it's the resistance that is quite tangible.

So, it's a total package that I have not seen put together before. And so, hearing you significant women and how you're dealing with life changes, life transitions, I believe it's going to be very effective, of high value for all those Boomer women, especially, that have hit the roadblocks or have hit this midlife—and sadly, many have no clue.

And so, I know a little bit about you. You were an editor at *Better Homes & Gardens*. Am I correct?

Cynthia: Yeah, I was a regional editor at *Better Homes*

& *Gardens* and *Traditional Home* for twenty years. That means I'm in the field, and what I do is, I would actually find the locations or go to designers and the artifacts—work with my photographer to photograph the location. Style them and write the article. So, I was a content editor.

Mitzi: Did you love it?

Cynthia: I did. I did. A lot of things came to change my path to what I'm doing right now, but I really loved it. It was great to have when my kids were little because every day I shot, I was away from home for two days working. I had the home office doing everything else. And so, I was able to raise my children and have a career at the same time. And make great money. So, it was really perfect for me.

Mitzi: Oh, and women would give their eyeteeth for those situations. How many children do you have?

Cynthia: Three.

Mitzi: And are they all leaving at this time?

Cynthia: Well, I've been crying all week. [Laughs]

Mitzi: Oh, your last one is gone?

Cynthia: No, it's not even that. They all went away. They all teamed up. I had boarding schools, home, college, home, the whole thing. And my eldest son got a job two months ago, and he came home right over the weekend and just packed up his car with everything he owns and he's gone. And the same day, my daughter moved out.

So, I had two gone in one day. I have one left, and he's going in a month. So, I'm having a very dead emptiness crisis going on here. And our house is not small but it's not big. It's only about 3800 square feet, but it feels really empty right now, and I'm not happy.

Mitzi: Oh, no. And I remember those days so well. And yeah, it's—there's nothing easy about it. I've always said and believe that those of us that love hard, hurt hard.

Cynthia: Yeah, true.

Mitzi: Basically, there are those of us that are really into it and enjoy and love our family and our kids, man, we hurt hard when all that's not there.

Cynthia: And the thing is I started—I never had my children until I was in my thirties. So I'm one of those typical Baby Boomers who waited longer than being in their twenties. I'm fifty-seven and I still have a twenty-one year old.

So, that's very typical of a lot of people my age or in our age group. So then the time does come for them to leave, and here we are, not like—my mom was forty-four when she was a grandmother. And so it's—

Mitzi: Oh, wow.

Cynthia: ...not like we're so young and we could start a career at forty-four. I think that a lot of people in our age group have maintained some kind of a business or career going forward when they had children. And if they didn't, those are the ones that are having a real crisis trying to get what they're going to do when they grow up. You know, they are fifty years old. And that's true, and also I find that those people who have never worked, and their kids are just going right now, are the ones that are having a harder adjustment than those of us who have worked all along. So, they're your audience that I will imagine is really going to be going through crisis.

Mitzi: Exactly. You're right, Cynthia, because they don't know which way to turn, and that's part of this whole process of the attitude and the mindset. "Okay, now what will I do?"

And so, what led you from what you were doing to The Daily Basics? And I'm just going to be kind of bold and ask you a question first, a caveat. Did you see the print lessening in its reach and saw the social media explosion, or was there something that moved you into what you're doing now?

Cynthia: Okay. So, you just answered half of my question—my answer, yes. My job as a magazine editor was to find trends before they became trends. I was always the first one on to digital, got into social media, into online...on to everything. And when I saw my magazines dropping off one by one—*Better Homes & Gardens* had 125 publications that we worked for and there were about forty of us who worked on a regular basis and made a great living. All of a sudden, the magazines dropped, and I called it Black Tuesday because every other Tuesday they were closing a magazine. And all the time there were some issues and they weren't accepting any jobs. And we got paid for the job. We were in contract.

So, it was definitely, you know, looking ahead and

Attitudes

saying we're going down fast. Here's the *Titanic*, and we're sinking, and over the last few years—I mean, I was the one who actually went to my editors and said, "Guys, you got to get involved in social media." And they are the ones that came out to a lot of my tweet ups and my in-real-life events to figure out what the progress was all about.

So, I've always been a promoter for doing that. So, yes, I rather saw the writing on the wall coming. I actually started thinking about The Daily Basics five years ago, and I think four years ago is when we launched.

So, it's been a real road of discovery because as far as blogging is concerned or websites are concerned, this was still in 1920s radio, as far as development was concerned. Everything has changed. People could do anything they wanted. It's brand new, and we're creating a new task. So that's the exciting part of doing this.

The reason that brought me into doing this was 9/11. We lived in New York. My husband loves to sail. And he came back from sailing up here in Newport, and he's part of a division in National Championships. And so, I really did not love living in Long Island at that point. I really didn't like it. It was getting crowded. And I had wanted to move for a long time. And he came home and he said he wanted to move on Monday, and on Tuesday, it was 9/11. And I said, you know something? We're so out of here. You know, Long Island is going down. New York is being hit. It's going to happen. We got to do something. So we left. After two years, we probably got it together. And we just picked up roots and moved to a place where we didn't know anyone at all. And that's what took us to Rhode Island. But we really wanted to eventually move, and we were at a good Baby Boomer point. We really wanted to eventually not live in Long Island, but where do we want to "retire"?

But I don't think there are a lot of us who will ever really retire—

Mitzi: No.

Cynthia: ...the way that we want to live. We decided we really—we're sailors. We wanted to live up in New England. Newport is an absolutely incredible town all year round, not just for summer months, and we've thought that this is where we wanted to be for the rest of our lives. So it's been a bit of a lifestyle change, which is what we wanted. But my husband still works in Manhattan and he goes there one day a week, and he has his own home office here. It's a four-hour commute one way.

Mitzi: Wow.

Cynthia: And I was just in New York for the last three days; I just got back last night. So, we hop on a plane. We hop on a train. We do more traveling than we did before, but it's a better lifestyle for us, and the kids have grown up a lot healthier. That's why I think a lot of people who have kids in their thirties and forties have to realize that they got to find where they want to live for the rest—you know "retire" when they're raising their kids. And don't live in a place that you hate because it's not worth it.

Mitzi: No, and that is about the attitude. You hit it right on the head, Cynthia, because so many people think they have no choice, that this is where it is and this is how my life is whether it works or not. And that's just not true. I mean, unless there's a really hardcore circumstance. But the majority of people do have a choice.

Attitudes

And it's actually very comforting for some Boomers to think they don't have a choice. If you believe that this is where you have to be, then you don't have to make a decision. But it takes a lot of courage to step up and do what you and your husband did.

It's easier to stay and complain and just go through the motions rather than start this whole matter of an emotional, physical process that actually changes everything. That's the inspiration that people want to hear and know it's doable. They can see and say "look at those people. They did it. We don't have to stay here and just make do. We can delve into another life somewhere, which is exactly what you did.

Cynthia: Right. It was very frightening, and at that time my mother was dying, she was struck with myeloma, which is the cancer of the blood. And so, I had taken care of her for eight years. And I said to my father, "You know, we got to get the kids up to move in toward the beginning of, you know, certain grades." And I'd come home every week. I'd come back and mom would come up and stay with me. And so, I left, and she died six months later. So, it was—

Mitzi: Wow.

Cynthia: ...an appropriate timing on that part, but I had to leave a dying mother, which was the hardest thing for me to do because I was very close to my mother. But I knew I had to do something for my family. So, you have to also put things in priority. And—

Mitzi: Good point.

Cynthia: ...and that was something that we did. It was

very difficult, but, you know what? I'm just sorry that we didn't do it sooner, when the kids were really little, you know? It's such a great life change.

Mitzi: Yeah. We all have to get to that point, but at least some of us get to that point. I mean, there are so many people who just accept what they really don't have to accept. So, I think you've answered question two, Cynthia. How did you set—how did you hit your personal reset button, explaining about the dropping off and Black Tuesday in the magazine world and just not liking where you were living and all, and then 9/11, of course. Was there anything else that was involved in you saying, "Okay, this is it here. We're totally moving, changing careers, moving location."

Cynthia: I think the decline of the magazines was a big thing. And even though I did work when I was up here—and I still actually do work for the magazines on a very, very minimal basis—it's just, I think, at that point in my life, I'd been doing it for so long. It's a lot of driving. I mean, when you go for a shoot, it's a lot of work, glamorous as it sounds, it is a lot of work.

And at that point I was in my fifties. I thought, I don't think I want to retire, but I've got to take my knowledge. And now that you've done something even if you were a housewife and did tremendous volunteer work, all of that is experience you could take and pull right into your next adventure, whether again it is a paid position or not. So, all these gals would think they had nothing going for them, but they were in the junior league or they were part of the PTA or they did this food bank. They got so much going on for them, and I always believe that is true for these women.

It's true, and I always think why can't we have a mom

who had five kids in the White House because she would turn this country around in two seconds. Those experiences are so valuable.

Yes. I mean, women really are, you know, very successful, multitaskers, and I think that's a really big point that I keep on drumming home to a lot of people who ask me, "You know, gee, where you been working all this time? You haven't stopped when you had kids, and you know I can't do it," but I'm sorry, but you really can do anything you want. And just seeing that gal who was sixty-four who swam from Cuba to Florida: you're never too old.

Yeah, it's just that there are so many great things about being this age at this time in history. I know that you're in your sixties, I'm in my fifties. I had lunch yesterday in New York with my two aunts. One is eighty-six, one is ninety, and they're both still working, and one has—

Mitzi: I love it!

Cynthia: ...traveled the world. Yup.

Mitzi: I love it. I love it.

Cynthia: Yeah.

Mitzi: That's going to be us, Cynthia.

Cynthia: That is going to be us, and that's going to be people who are thinking in that attitude range that there's no reason why you have to stop. No reason.

Why? You're going to retire and sit home and play scrabble all day long? No. Not happening. That's—no, no or shop or whatever you do. No, I won't do that. I hate shopping. No, I'm not doing it.

And I also swim, and I have a bunch of gals that swim with me who are in their seventies and eighties and they swim one to two miles at a time.

Mitzi: Oh, yeah. There you go. It's all the total package. It's taking care of yourself. It's taking care of your home, your environment. It's everything, and we can't isolate. The point of this is that one factor is not going to catapult us into the Boomer years or the later years that we're all wanting and deserving. It's the whole enchilada, so to speak. I mean, you just touched on the big point, and that is taking the time to take care of yourself. It's obviously critical, but it's amazing for women, how they put themselves behind everything else. And, "Oh, when I have time, I will exercise," or "When I have time, I will start doing whatever." There's never going to be time. I mean, it just has—

Cynthia: No.

Mitzi: ...to be priority. I wrote somewhere that Boomers, when they get to their fifties and especially their sixties, are a walking billboard of what they did in their forties and early fifties. We're not doomed or resilient at turning things around, and it's like you said, it's never too late for anything. But there are consequences to not taking care of ourselves. And we have to do that in order to have the stamina and the health and the energy to do these new things.

So, they're definitely connected. And I love what you said about using your knowledge and not wanting to work so hard on something that is out of your season. I mean, you did that. We were excellent at it, at your "season" with the magazines. It's over. Now, what am I going to do? And I feel that way about my interior design. It's hard work, like you said, and as a thirty-year professional designer who hears, "Oh, Mitzi, I would love to have your job, it looks like it's so much fun." They have no idea how hard it is.

Cynthia: No. They do not know how hard we worked behind the scenes.

Mitzi: And I don't want to do that. I'm sixty-seven now. I'm the oldest of the Baby Boomers, and I love design. It's in my blood. It's like you're still doing the writing and everything, but my ideal is to do like one or two clients at a time, maybe, and the rest be giving back, doing the teaching and the writing and teaching CEUs and that kind of speaking.

So did you know you were getting to this? That you were going to leave the magazine at some point before the social media, Daily Basics boot camp was birthed, or did this—

Cynthia: Who knew that the Internet was going to take over the information network? I mean, I felt that I'd be doing this forever. I love my job, and I thought, our kids will be older and I'll be able to really have a great career going forward. My mentor taught me everything I know in the magazine business; she is seventy-eight and she still shoots. And she's still the New York editor for *Traditional Home*. Her name is Bonnie Maharam. She's amazing.

So she's out there shooting, and we have another one, that girl who's over in Boston. She's still shooting. She's almost ninety. I mean, these gals are always out there. So, we do have magazines still going forward, but it's been a big change, and I think a lot of my other—

I called them my other mentors—who are around the country have all segued into secondary, into tertiary projects besides the H&G or TradHome, and it really is—now you could do, I think, those combos. Who knew that that was all going to happen, and that's the point. You never know what your future holds or where technology is going, but the most important thing is if you see something that could be pertinent to what you're doing, hop on the train and don't be afraid to explore social media.

Here I am, fifty-seven years old; I'm not even close to knowing it all. But I'm totally engaged because, from experience, I know all about this stuff, and the only reason I can is because I'm not scared to look at this. So it's not something so smart—it's to say I'm not scared.

Mitzi: Well, you were so encouraging to meet, Cynthia, because at sixty-five, you know, I was practically signing up for Medicare when I was getting into social media and blogging, etc. It sounds so ancient. But the reality is I was starting social media at that point, and of course, everyone I'm around is younger than my kids. And so, to overcome the—I guess embarrassment and maybe even sharing that oh, my gosh, I just—no, I can't figure this stuff out. Why don't I know this? Why can't I get this?

There's that overcoming that has to occur in order to get to what is next for us. Most of the time it's not going to be this easy hand in our lap: "Oh, here you go, Cynthia," "Here it is, Mitzi." There is a calculated effort, don't you think? I mean, for that challenge, if it is going to be something that is fulfilling.

Cynthia: Yeah, and I think there's nothing—I mean, every time I go to a new, you know, real-life event or tweet up, I am always thrilled to see that most of the people are over forty, and the ones that are the younger ones are actually really not getting the power of social media. They go to school and they're learning communication and they say, "This is how Twitter works. But that's the best thing of being at this point in our lives and understanding what our original content is that we had developed over the years of our own careers, and if you could just get into the social media, you will find that you are the king of the hill because not only do you know how to tweet but you know how to put the real information out there.

Mitzi: I love that—

Cynthia: It's true. It's just so great being this age and knowing the technical. You know the old saying—oh gosh, I'm going to forget how it goes but—well, it's actually, it's called youth displacement, but the whole premise is if you had known what you did when you were twenty, you'd be so much better off. Well, I do know what the twenty year olds are knowing right now. I know the social media. So, I am able to take that and mix it in with young stuff and play it to my experience. So, I feel like I'm in my twenties. So, it's good. It's really good stuff.

Mitzi: It's awesome to hear that youth in your voice, Cynthia, and the passion that you have, and how blessed and fortunate you are to move into this arena that will take you into Foreverville. I feel the same way about design. I love design. I can't imagine my world without being—having a pulse somewhere into it. I love my clients, most of them, but that's not all I can do right now. I have to pursue this.

Okay, last question is—and you touched on it many times, but I didn't cover something you would like to say, is what is working best about this new path you are on? What is so good about it?

Cynthia: It's—you know what? Everything. It's exciting. It's a new adventure. It's a new life. I'm traveling more. The potential to make money is so huge if you could, you know, get yourself into the right hookups. So, I'm working on actually monetizing The Daily Basics through working with companies and connecting with social media and bloggers in various ways. So, I've actually gone out of my own comfort zone by doing that. So, that, yeah, that's not my field. I mean, I'm not—that's not what I do, but it is now. So, that's been great. My husband is so supportive and he is such an angel. So, he's getting kind of excited about this because…like we just got back from Italy in July. We were there for the launch of the testing of some wines that we were, you know, helping them promote to our social media group. And so, they got to go with me. So, we ended up being in Italy for ten days and having a blast. It's an adventure, and that is, I think, the most exciting thing, you know, the world is still my oyster. It could be anybody's oyster, I think, engaging upon something to explore. You do have to take care of yourself. Maintenance is key. Maintenance for your husband is key. So, if you want to have your mate around for a while, you make sure they go for their checkups and they do what I call maintenance things. So something is wrong? You try to fix it or adjust it or learn how to live with this.

Mitzi: Exactly.

Cynthia: That health thing is really, really important,

but going forward, it's just nothing but exciting. So, that's, I think, what will keep us younger. I also think being a mother of twenty somethings who will be having grandchildren one day and raising them, I'm their role model. My husband is a role model, and if you cannot show your children how it is that you are living, then they will not know that they have to go forward and do the same thing with their life and pass that—I did get this so from my mother who was an interior designer. I worked for her for five years.

Mitzi: Oh, really?

Cynthia: Yeah, so this is how I know this business. And she unfortunately dealt with myeloma when she was sixty-six. But she wasn't willing to stop. She actually was—she had eight years of the cancer, and for four years going into it, when she was really sick, she would not stop working. And she did it with dignity, and she always had her makeup on and she always was fabulous, and she was always in New York and always doing and doing. So, your role models are very important but it's important for you to be the role model. That's what you're doing for your children as well. And also for your boys. Who are they going to marry? And your grandson, who will he have? You know, they're going to see that their grandmother was out there, you know, kicking butt and doing all these great things because they want to live like that, you know? [Laughs]

Mitzi: Yes, exactly. Somebody did mention in one of the interviews that our kids, our grown kids, want to see us happy, whatever that looks like, and their lives are going to be really busy, and that's the way it's supposed to be. They're busy living and growing up and raising family and they want mom and dad to be doing their thing so that they can do their thing. And it's around that, that way of saying what you just said, that we're not to be one that is pitied and home, and, "Oh, I got to call my mother. I haven't talked to her for three days and I don't—and she's just so lonely and she's this and that." We're not those women, and our children are blessed because we never will be those women no matter what. And so that was an excellent point you brought up. Cynthia? What advice would you give other Boomers debating over what to do when their future plans have not worked out the way they thought?

Cynthia: Their future plans are not going to work out the way they want, there's no question about it.

Mitzi: Excellent point. That's life. That's life. You know, when things happen in life and everybody is just so upset and they can't go forward and there's too much to handle, well, pick yourself up—put your big girl panties on and go forward because that's life. And if you can't handle it, then you're going to be missing out. So, what are you going to do when things don't work out? You take stuff out. I'm a big risk taker. I make sure that everything fits or is right.

Cynthia: So, make a list of everything, all that you have done that you loved and everything that you've done that you hated. And start looking at things that you'd like to do that really focus around the things that you loved, and if there's something that you really hate, might as well knock that off the list, like working in an office. I hated that. So, that's off my list.

Mitzi: **Right.**

Attitudes

Cynthia: So just pull out the positive, in other words, from your life and look for things that you think you would like to do in those arenas. I think everybody—they were also coming from a very weird kind of time period where everybody felt entitled, and as parents, we had given our children too much and our kids are entitled. And we are not only the culprits but it's a society culprit that has been at play here.

Mitzi: Right.

Cynthia: My daughter will say, "But I want to be in my career. I want to be happy." I'm like, "You can't be. You got to work for it. Pay your dues. Stop crying. Pick yourself up and go." And it's the same advice I would give anybody who's in their fifties and sixties who wanted to do something new. You know, if you want to go and travel the world and write a travel book, figure out your finances. Sell your house. Go on a boat. You know, take an RV across—I mean, do whatever you need to make it happen. You *can* make it happen. But stop crying about it and lamenting and just go forward. So that's my answer. It's not going to work out. Just figure it out.

Mitzi: I love when you so profoundly said, "Well, it won't work out." I mean that is so profound, Cynthia, because how many people have a plan with downsizing jobs and just everything happening differently from what our parents have? I mean, what we're experiencing. Things aren't going to be the same.

Cynthia: My mother's favorite movie was *Moonstruck* and when Cher said, you know, "Knock it off; get over it." And that was her favorite thing. Even when she was so sick, she would say, "Get over it. Knock it off. Go forward." But it's really—it's a changing world, and you know, we're in a very bad financial time right now.

Mitzi: Right.

Cynthia: I think people have just about had it, you know; be positive and adjust and go forward. And there's nothing more you can do than that. And you know, it's life. It's life, but if you want it, you know, you do it. If you feel like giving up and watching daytime TV all the time, go ahead. Have a good time. But that's not who we are and that's not who our generation is, I don't think, I really don't. It's been great talking to you, and I'm really excited about reading this book. It sounds terrific. You inspire me.

Mitzi: Thank you. And this is the journey that we're on, reaching out to others when we're doing things that we love and we're wanting to have others love what they're doing. I mean, it bothers us when we see people with lots of potential. It's such a lose-lose versus the win-win. You know, they lose and people around them, our society, loses when they're stuck and they don't open up their attitudes like we've been talking about.

So, the whole key is this attitude mindset, and I think we would be shocked if we knew that hundreds and thousands, probably millions of Boomers, are literally stuck, Cynthia, and think they have no choices. And so, we're not going to reach everybody, but those that have ears to hear and eyes to see that there's another way—I'm excited that we might have an impact on them.

Cynthia: Well, I think you are doing this at a very appropriate time because seventy-percent of the women in

Attitudes

this country are single, and they are looking for—

Mitzi: I thought it was fifty-percent. You've heard a statistic that says seventy?

Cynthia: I've heard seventy percent. And so that fact alone, they're sitting at home or looking for the husband, the next husband. And I got news for you. You can't waste your life looking for a husband. You got to do your own thing, and then you'll meet your husband. And I think that that's why this book is really impactful. You got to show women that they can't just be looking for love in one arena; when you find your passion of doing something else, it will fulfill you, and then you'll find people who are interested in what you're doing.

So, for that, she has to be in a place where she's meeting her other needs. The whole purpose that motivates women out of where they are because they need to be doing more for themselves.

And so, that financial is a big thing, and learning to be satisfied with less, learning to find yourself, and it's exactly what you said. It's not all about a husband, that's for sure. Many married women wish they were single. That's so true. You know, I think that you and I are probably some of the very few who have great marriages or have, you know, a stable home and environment. I consider myself very lucky, but most—not most, I'd say a good portion of my friends are not happy, and they're always complaining about their spouse or they're single and complaining about not having a spouse. So, go find your own path and go down it, and whatever that may be, go find yourself and find out who you are. And that's just the path to go on. But it's really about what you're talking about, the whole person, taking care of yourself, and if you're happy with who you are, you're going to be happy in general no matter what.

Mitzi: Well said. Well, thank you, Cynthia; and we'll be in touch and I can't...I can't thank you enough.

Cynthia: Okay, love. Thank you. I'm so glad you thought of me. Thank you. I'm very honored by the way. Thank you.

Barbara Barton
Barbara Barton & Associates
www.BarbaraBarton.net

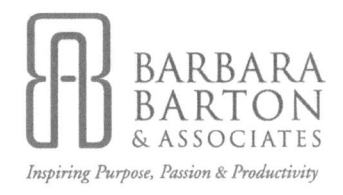

BARBARA BARTON & ASSOCIATES
Inspiring Purpose, Passion & Productivity

Mitzi: Well, I so appreciate you doing this, Barbara. I've had the most enlightening conversations with women across the country, and I'll tell you what, there's just a whole lot that the Boomers have to say about this whole aging thing and what they think about it. So, I'm anxious to hear what you have to say. But you and I have this history of talking about preparing for aging. Certainly, you're one that's even thinking about it.

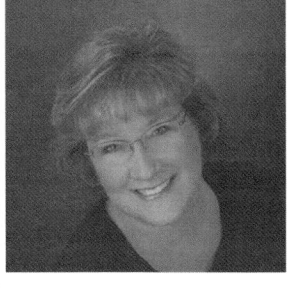

So, your chapter is Attitude. And this chapter is promoting aging with Boomer Smarts in attitude. One part of it is what we are putting in our thinking, whether it is positive or negative as garbage in, garbage out. We Boomers get to choose what our thoughts on aging are. Where our thinking goes, we go. It is thought that controls are behaviors.

Another facet of the garbage in and garbage out theory is, basically, who we associate with and what's going on around us. Are we receiving what they're saying or not? Do we have a discerning mindset attitude on what other Boomers are thinking, saying, and doing? And that's really a very critical part. So many Boomers naively respond, "Well, everybody is doing this," or "nobody else is doing blah blah blah."

Well then let's hit it. The first one is what do you want to change in your current attitude position by choosing whether it would be your lifestyle, your housing, your work schedule, social, whatever it might be? What comes to mind when that question is posted to you?

Barbara: I'm just going to share with you what those first thoughts were, the keyword in this question is "choosing." So, even being asked "what are you wanting to choose to change in your life?" I had to look at a lot of aspects. Number one, I'm single. So, I even went through the whole process. Do I choose to have a partner with me in this next chapter? And it didn't really resonate—didn't rise to the top—but these things did. The one thing that I really want to choose is flexibility with a capital F in time management. And this is including healthy living choices. So, moving in to more exercise or moving in to more reading...It made me stop and think that, number one, I even have a choice. It's reminding me that I have a choice. And to look at every aspect and see which ones I really do want to change.

Now, three years ago, I made a choice about my housing and, as a person who already fell downstairs in her town home, I believe that the only thing I could do to take care of that aspect, which is really key to me, assuming that I'm a designer and when I have designed many homes and help people nurture each other, my new home hasn't nurtured me.

Mitzi: Well said.

Barbara: So, I chose an adult community condominium; three-story with an elevator facing a golf course. I don't give a flip about golf. But it felt like, it felt like I have a backyard that has ducks and reminds me of how precious nature is. I live in a ranch-style condo. I've always known that I'm that kind of a housing person.

So, I was really gratified to know that even my thinking three years ago at age sixty-one was important. And I'm still living with it.

Mitzi: Before you had the accident falling down the steps, had you given any thought to your physical needs in your spaces, or did it come about after the wake-up call?

Barbara: I had given thought to it, like I was saying. I realized that I'm a condo person. I'm not the kind that wants to fret with the gardens. And I've been single. I've been single for, gosh, let's see, about forty years.

So, being single, I knew that I had to be the one that took the initiative.

And I work. I wasn't doing it for anyone else. That could either be helpful or not, but anyway, it works. It works.

Mitzi: I'm working with so many women throughout this endeavor and on social media who are single. It's astounding to me, and so we looked at the demographics of the Boomers, and my goodness…where is our reality check? I'm just still shocked at the statistics from the last census.

Also that the demographics have almost flipped upside down between what they call "American family," what single-family housing looks like, and the whole housing "normal" is not normal anymore. It's so totally skewed in what most of us perceive is really going on in America. And it's just been such an eye-opener to me how many women are just like you. And I think of the women I'm talking to as the movers and shakers, like you. I picked you all because I want you to be the examples and inspire other people with your successes and also with what you know is—I don't know if vulnerability is the right word—but just the necessity of moving in a different direction. You know what I'm saying?

And so, it's just been amazing to me that this group of women in their fifties and sixties are coming up on some critical life-changing choices and we're not talking about it. I don't hear a lot of dialogue about single women, what Boomer women are going to do, and any one of us could be single at any time. We all know women that have been married forever, and their husbands say, "Oh, by the way, I don't want to be married anymore," and their life is turned upside down and for certain not so predictable any more—not to mention all those Boomers losing a spouse to sickness or accidents, etc.

With that said, you've already answered about the flexibility and wanting to choose to have more time for you. What is your attitude regarding your own aging? There are really two different questions. This one being: are you content with where you are and why? What is good and what is not so good? And I know it's about not having the flexibility, but beyond that, what is working for you, Barbara, and what is not?

Barbara: Well, when I really looked hard at that, I realized that, internally, I'm thirty-five. Internally, that was my pitch year in my life. I was on top of everything in the world. Externally, there is an attitude that has grown, especially in the last six months, because I've had to face what physical aging has done. And how my attitude could affect my vulnerability.

So, accepting what does not work and what does work with my physical well-being then could spill into the mental and emotional. But the physical is the biggest challenge.

And if I were to say that what is working, what is good, is that I have ended up surrendering to the wonderful professional healthcare workers that are helping me on my behalf. This has been an attitude adjustment from absolute frustration and desperation on what it was that I could do to change myself physically to surrendering to the fact that I have helpers.

Mitzi: Okay. So, what are they to you?

Barbara: They are part of my team.

Mitzi: Okay. I think I know that what you mean is that it's not about you figuring it out and going your own way and "I'm fine, thank you very much" to "okay, I need to know what you guys know and let's work together." Am I hearing you right?

Barbara: That is still just one aspect, however. The word advocacy still pops up. And the advocacy has to start with me and in my acceptance of my own responsibility in finding out what aspects I can do and then being able to be a partner in the decisions and the questions and follow it through. I will tell you it leads to one of the not-so-good, which is—it leads to feeling overwhelmed.

Mitzi: Yes, okay.

Barbara: I mean, if people could quit sending me ten direct mail items a day on how am I going to correct high blood pressure, my weight issue, and lose natural whatever on the market, to even getting all of my very well-meaning friends who are suggesting, "Why don't you see this person and that person and this person and that person?" It's overwhelming. You have abundance of health—that's great. At the same time, it could be overwhelming.

So, what else is working? Well, what I'm discovering, especially this year, financially, is that I am living more simply. I'm embracing the fact that living more simply oftentimes means I don't have to hurry everywhere. I don't have to push myself so much. And I will say this is, this is my warmer side. When a friend of mine was facing his death, one of the comments that he made to me was, "Why is everybody in such a hurry?" And I felt like this was a very straight-up observation, especially coming out of desperation. So, whether you're slowing the pace and really able to understand more internal peace. So, what's working for me is my faith.

Mitzi: Beautiful.

Barbara: And my...and my reading time, my private time. But I still have a list of what's not working, too.

Mitzi: Well, I'm sure, and if you're—if you feel like sharing some of those, that would be good, too, Barbara. But I would only want you to share what you feel like. I mean, this is not to pry, it's just to help others.

Barbara: Yeah, of course it is. And the whole process that you've taken me through is very eye-opening and very supportive. So, I made a list of what is not working as well, is paying for the lack of focus on my physical health. I'm paying for that now, whether that's playing catchup, whether that's educating on what my body needs. Another big area that's not working, that I had tended to push aside for the sake of a professional mentality (I thought I was going to go ahead and die at my desk), is the lack of hobbies or playtime. What is it that I can help create outside of my profession and help me…that gives me a new sense of joy? I know it's out there, but I haven't yet discovered exactly what that looks like.

Mitzi: Yes, for sure. That's a huge thought right there because, as type A personalities, we always have something else out there ahead of what we're thinking or doing, and that is a big part of living life—the balance. And I'm hearing that a lot from many of us Boomers.

Barbara: I know.

Mitzi: Yeah. It is so easy to have our life be in a professional status, even our social connections. And I think that's where you're saying you would like to change, to do some things that are separate from that; even though we have friends, you know, there's no—there's still ramifications or consequences if we don't do whatever everyone else expects us to do.

And having relationships or hobbies, or whatever it

Attitudes

might look like that separates us from our professional life, is very healthy. And I've seen that, Barbara. I mean that's really wisdom.

Barbara: And so, what I realized in this exercise is that what it takes is what I will call shoring up your attitude, since you're focusing the chapter about attitude. How is it that I can shore it up? How is it that I can take one small step to commit to a social group that would allow me growth and step forward outside of my profession? This is new.

Mitzi: Cool.

Barbara: This requires some courage from me, and requires some inspiration.

Mitzi: Yeah, that requires courage to find them and go out and do it, you know. Are you thinking of anything in particular? If you could do what you wanted to do, Barbara, with some sweet time, what would give you that joy? I mean, those are the things you're probably thinking about, and maybe they're tied together to getting your health in order. But even while you're pondering this, and by the way, I believe you're going to be extremely successful. I just know it. Just your personality. Once you decide, once you make that choice, you are already mentally and emotionally ready to go for it, Barbara.

Barbara: I appreciate it.

Mitzi: Oh, yeah. No, I'm a good judge of character, Barbara, and you're not just going to roll over and let aging happen.

Barbara: Yeah.

Mitzi: That's not going to happen, but when you talked about how you felt about your own aging, thirty-five inside, what was joyful about that? Is that a part of your—

Barbara: I think it ties in to this question. As a career coach, what I realized is that I am doing what I love to do, and there is an adage that I learned many, many, many, years ago and I believe it. And that is that people—all they ever wanted to do in their life is to contribute, especially to another human being.

There is nothing that drives people more. So, when I work at what's missing, I have that in my profession as a career coach. What's still underneath that is what I knew my passion was when I was a teenager. And that was creating nurturing homes for everyone.

So, when I look at where I can contribute—I'm going to have a Habitat for Humanity endeavor of some sort, hopefully. So I contribute money where that passion touches my heart.

Mitzi: Beautiful.

Barbara: Where I think that comes into play is they still need volunteers, and they don't need volunteers just to swing a hammer.

So, the whole realm of "follow your passion," being around people who believe in the same concept, the same cause, that is where I think I'm missing out a lot, not giving myself the social time, the playing time for the heart.

Mitzi: Yes, and as females, especially, we just have to

have that to thrive. I think it is the most for men, too, but they don't require the relationship, nurturing, communication that we women do and it—it is absolutely essential. And when I was asking another special interviewer, her name is Doreen Hanna and she's in California, she started Modern Day Princesses, which mentors teenagers. She said once she was over that with her own children, she never thought she would be going back to being involved with teenage girls. But it led to a women's ministry and has moved into helping younger women. And so, she and I were discussing how women—she's our age, give or take a couple of years, in her sixties, also. And we were discussing how many women we know that feel so isolated or so purposeless and lonely; even when they're with people, if they're not doing like what you were just discussing. And how we can encourage ourselves also, but these other women, they don't have to still be working or they may never have worked. But the point is they're within themselves. They're not looking outward.

And when you talked of these words, of basic human need, if you contribute, that's got to be the antidote to the isolation and depression and loneliness. I mean it's not like the magic bullet, but it certainly is a huge antidote. And so, what choices do you need to make now to accelerate them, to prepare for your personal future? You've identified what the need is in areas that you want to rework, so to speak; is this all so fresh and just occurring now for you to consider it? Or have you gone to the next level yet to think about—I mean, besides your physical therapy and your team, your advocates. But what about the other parts of your life? Have you started to consider any of those yet?

Barbara: I'm glad that you post it in the realm of it being a choice. That's very empowering. You asked the question "are you content?" No, I am not content. Am I adjusting? I'm in the process of adjusting. So, the choices: one choice is to be okay with my financial decisions. That's the first one. And I'm fortunate enough to embrace self-employment because that's the ability to show that I have many different hats I can wear, that it doesn't have to be one thing like I thought it was. The second thing is I'm measuring a new definition of life success.

So, there's this old quote about what success really means. I can't even think who it is or what it is, but I remember the impression, and this is probably the gift that wisdom gives us as long as we can remember. And that is that the measurement of success in this contribution—and there is an underlying acceptance in success. And that is, you have to be accepting of your own mistakes.

I've had to embrace, this is part of an attitude adjustment, and I'm a newbie. I'm a newbie at something. And if I am stretching myself for new choices, I've got to be willing to fall on my face. I've got to be willing to be embarrassed. I've got to be willing to face that I'm going to make some bad choices and some mistakes. I call it making mistakes with grace.

Mitzi: Oh, I love that. That's beautiful. That should be on a pillow.

Barbara: I think so, too. So, at the serious things—All right. I have to remember that I have experiences to choose to rely on to keep me moving forward. In other words, I don't have to beat myself up for this falling on my face, for the embarrassing moment that happened when I was twenty-four, or for what appears to be a big hiccup in the road called divorce or any of that kind of crap. That I can still choose to remember the experiences that empower me forward. That's the choice.

And the last—you've actually already touched on it, and I think it's sort of the encapsulation of everything that you've heard from a lot of people, and that is how do we achieve balance more readily? We know that sometimes that when we're at peace, right, being able to have that balance from activity to peacefulness, from stimulation to agreement, and how it plays out.

Mitzi: Anticipating, isn't it? I mean, it's…it's all-encompassing about our wholeness in living a life of balance. That's well-said, Barbara, totally, and everybody is striving for that, and I—my personal reflection on that is every day is a new day on what that balance looks like and, of course, right now, that's kind of a joke for me. But it won't be that way forever, and I…I do control my life when I shut off and shut down.

And I have people that are in my life that look at me like I have three heads when I say, "You know, after 7 PM or whatever, I'm not online. I can't do all those things that I used to do ten years ago in the evening." And I'm very much okay with that, but a lot of other people aren't. I mean, they expect because we're in this being normal that we're all going to accept it too. And I can't physically and by my choices, I don't like or want to. No, I'm not doing that. But, if you could give one tip to fellow Baby Boomers, what would you say to them on preparing for their futures?

Barbara: Well, I can't narrow down to one but I can give you two.

Mitzi: Good.

Barbara: Probably the biggest thing that I've learned even answering these questions, but also in the last several months, is that I'm vulnerable but I'm not alone.

And the other thing that keeps me going with a good attitude is something that a friend gave me a long time ago just from some conversations, and this is what I call mirror talk.

You put on those affirmations or inspiring words on your mirror and every day you look at them and this one…this one has seemed to have carried me through the good times and bad and, to a degree, and I can't say, you know, it holds me true a hundred percent every time, but the words are these: "I can do this." That's it.

Mitzi: I love it.

Barbara: Whatever I'm facing, whatever I'm feeling, I can do this.

Mitzi: That's profound, very, very—I've heard this from many people, and it's been around forever, but life is ten percent what happens to us and ninety percent how we respond to it.

We tell ourselves with our attitude, "Ah, no big deal, Mitzi. You can do this. I can do this."

Barbara: Uh huh.

Mitzi: Well, just knowing that you can do this and you're working on it, takes you from the realm of "holy crap, what am I going to do now," which of course is always often our first response when something is identified or happens. But you've taken the bull by the

Attitudes

horns, so to speak, and you have your team. You are working on it. By your behavior, you're saying, "I can do this. I will do this."

And that's huge, Barbara, that's just a really big deal because the flip side to that is, "Oh, man. Is this the beginning of la-la-la-la-la?" And of course, that's a normal reaction also, but it's a position of being the victim rather than fighting. And one of the whole points of doing this, for me, is to encourage, inspire, and educate Boomers to fight with the Boomer Smart Attitude.

I loved the ending to the question saying, "I can do," and that's a way of saying, "I'm fighting this. I'm going to fight whatever. I'm not going to roll over and just accept all this and age negativity like everybody else."

Barbara: Right. I'm going to suggest to you when I hear you talk about how you can pull yourselves up by your bootstraps and go ahead and fight it, I've learned in a lot of self-empowerment seminars and stuff like that in we try to resist what's so that we actually create more suffering, but if we can accept and embrace, and you just have to make about the word embrace, that means hugging it. That means kissing it. That means actually saying, "This is a part of what I'm feeling." And all of a sudden after that embrace, it goes away. Whatever we resist, persist. This is coming from the Sedona Method, and that Sedona Method of releasing our resistances to everything that's happened to us is probably one of the biggest peace pills earned.

Mitzi: And the happiest people are the ones that are satisfied and that are contributing. And that's one of the things I see in America as far as where we're headed as a country, is that there is so much inwardness. And if we can draw Boomers out. I've always told you this,

I have maybe or maybe not, but it's for those Boomers that have ears to hear and eyes to see and a mind and a heart to get it. That's going to be big because there are people out there that are not hearing the voices that we've been talking about, our internal subconscious, and really getting still with themselves and starting to evaluate this, examining our futures and what it may look like. We just push it aside, don't process any of it in our busyness.

And so, it's a big, big, dimension, this attitude, and that's why I spent two chapters, one on mindset and then followed up by attitudes. And it's like what good is it to learn about any of the other things that we know are important if you're closed-minded, if you're unteachable?

So, what I've heard from you, Barbara, in this time of your interview, is that your mind is open and you are definitely thinking. Of course, you're very teachable and I just applaud where you are, Barbara. And I respect you tremendously and it's an honor to be in your circle.

Barbara: Oh, thank you, Mitzi. You've got such a generous heart and I appreciate the acknowledgment, you don't know. And—

Mitzi: Thank you.

Barbara: ...even the process of going through this was a gift.

Chapter 4
Routines

Boomer Smarts: Healthy Aging Is
75% Lifestyle, 25% Genetics

Baby Boomers Will Transform Aging in America, Panel Says —Huffington Post March 15, 2013

Big news...Have you heard it? There is a major tsunami coming! And we even know where it is going to hit—it is going to hit very soon in America!

There is already a name for this tsunami that is about to crash in on our country.

It is called the Silver Tsunami!

According to a panel of experts at the Aging in America Conference on April 1, 2013, we Boomers face both opportunities and potential crises.

By 2020, the population of Americans age 55 to 65 will have grown an unprecedented 73% since 2000. Ken Dychtwald of Age Wave says, "Anyone who thinks the boomers will turn 65 and be the same as the generation before are missing out on the last 60 years of sociology. The boomers change every stage of life through which they migrate."

Of course we know why—there are 78 million Boomers! But do we or have we even begun to grasp the ramifications of this huge phenomenon already nipping away at our shores?

Most definitely not!

We Boomers will and are putting a huge strain on entitlement programs like Social Security benefits and Medicare. In 2010, 39 million Americans received Social Security benefits, and this was before the oldest of the Boomers turned sixty-five and was eligible and mandated to receive Medicare benefits.

And by 2020, 64 million people will be eligible for Medicare, a whopping one-third more than today. Do the math! Do we have that many in the younger generations coming up the ranks to participate and contribute working capital into these systems? Census takers reveal a big "no," since many will be minorities trying to achieve a higher standard of living as our American landscape changes. This is not a political commentary but pure mathematical data that affects all Boomers RIGHT NOW.

I just feel so strongly and so passionately the absolute necessity of getting these facts known to this huge Baby Boomer demographic that will be affected in their health care benefits beyond what any of the experts can possibly predict. Sadly for us Boomers, however, is the certainty that it will not be pretty.

Chronic disease is the single biggest driver of health care costs, says Dr. Rhonda Randall, chief medical officer of United Healthcare, and sixty percent of those over sixty-five live with one or more chronic diseases, such as diabetes and heart disease.

Dr. Randall says that insurers are working to better coordinate care so that seniors stay healthy longer. I say and believe that is a good thing, but we Boomers need to be the ones trying to stay healthier longer by our lifestyle Routine.

Our lifestyle Routine is very simply our only possible hope for securing a better health future...not our genetic background. Research doctors and experts no longer believe a genetic predisposition to be an inevitability in our future health.

And I can hear the shouts already about how such predispositions as the cancer gene are part of our genetic makeup. Of course this is understood and assumed. But the lifestyle effect on our health cannot be disputed... especially since well over thirty percent of Americans are not only considered overweight but obese.

To go into any battle one must know the enemy. Baby Boomers equipped with Boomer Smarts know their enemy and it has a name: apathy. However, these Boomers with Boomer Smarts will slay this enemy by not only caring about their future health but actually learning what to do and then doing it with all the Boomer gusto they can muster up to fight and fight hard to keep their Boomer health.

My Personal Silver Tsunami

My personal tsunami episode occurred with one phone call out of the blue. Arlene Evans-Debeverly, an exceptional PA-C and national expert in women's health issues, called me herself and said, "I want to see you in my office at eight o'clock tomorrow morning."

Now this was a "yikes" for sure! It takes months to get in to see Arlene, so that fact alone said something was up and it probably was not good news. And it wasn't.

Bob went with me to this appointment to hear Arlene say that if I fell off a bike or was injured in a car accident or any other of life's unplanned accidents, I could be in a wheelchair for the rest of my life. What??? Me???

I have been ultra dedicated in taking care of my health for many years, but obviously something was very wrong with my routine that was putting me at such risk. There is a name that the tests showed, and it is osteoporosis... the silent killer. And boy was it ever silent!

Now this was not my first bone density test, but at this age, my numbers took a dive from being osteopenia to the full-blown osteoporosis. Now my personal profile of being from an Eastern European background, small framed with light eyes and skin, and not taking hormone supplements during menopause of course contributed to my bone density report revealing the osteo. However, many, many women with just the opposite personal profiles are dealing with this condition also. Sadly, however, many either do not know or do not know how to fight it vigorously.

I cannot even express the importance and the power of seeing the right medical professional to obtain the proactive up-to-date treatments for whatever your health situations may be. Find them! Don't be a nice little Boomer that says "okay, give me the meds that everyone else is taking" without researching all Boomer options on any given health issue. Fight like your life depends on it because it does!

Suffice it to say that Arlene spent a lengthy time with Bob and me showing us models of bone and what happens in the good bone versus the bad bone, which was an incredible but scary demonstration of where my bones were and why she was so majorly concerned about my future health. Her knowledge and experience and expertise, however, were what saved my lifestyle routine for my future by explaining the most acceptable and most prescribed treatment. A trial period showed that this was not going to be aggressive enough for my osteo numbers to improve.

Enter Arlene's knowledge and experience and most of all, her heart and motivation to get me back to living my life without this scary threat of osteoporosis; she saved

Routines

me...literally! She explained and then prescribed very new medications most had not heard of yet. And we were on our way to getting Mitzi back to wholeness

My health battle was on big time! I was not going to just accept this and change my lifestyle to accommodate some stupid diagnosis. NO, NO, NO, NOT ME!

I sadly hear so many Boomers saying "my arthritis" or "my whatever" is acting up. Well, I say kick that "whatever" in the butt and do something about it!

I will never be convinced that there is never ever any hope and that a diagnosis is just a concrete decree that Boomers must accept as their bodies age. For Pete's sake, already...we are the Baby Boomers, remember? We changed everything forever, so why would we not rebel against the most important issue of our lives...our own Boomer health?

But I am hearing a thunderous sound across America that is getting louder and louder and louder, that is shouting, "No, not me! I can control my health by my daily lifestyle routine!"

And change my daily routine I certainly did by learning that eighty percent of Americans are deficient in Vitamin D, which is essential for calcium absorption. I took a very high prescribed amount of Vitamin D for three months and was tested again, showing my numbers had indeed climbed to the correct level.

But—and this is another big but, which includes my all-out-effort to gain my bone density to a healthier condition—what did this look like? Well, I researched all I could to learn what the latest-known facts on osteo were. I learned that drinking soda is a huge no no, smoking the number one no no, of course alcohol in excess, a high-salt diet, and not enough weight-bearing exercise. So even though most of these no nos weren't in my routine, being aware is the answer. There is tons of info on what to eat and what not to eat for treating this chronic condition that is a battle I will win.

After two years of medical treatments, supplements, specific exercises, and diet, along with my natural hormone replacement therapy, my bone density numbers were remarkably positive and my aggressive treatment was actually working! Wow, more proof to me that even if we have a bad report, we don't just talk about it, worry about it, or accept that report. We take the bull by the horns and believe that we will, of course, overcome high blood pressure, pre-diabetes, aches and pains from arthritis, and other conditions. How? by changing our routines and seeking Boomer Smarts from whatever source we can, and believe me, those sources are everywhere. Remember? We are in the information age, so lack of knowledge or lack of Boomer Smarts is simply not the Boomer way to fight back.

Obviously, these beliefs of mine and zillions of other Boomers who are now fighting hard to age better and age smarter in America are in no way meant for medical advice. Pure and simple, my only purpose is to wake up the already savvy Baby Boomers to arm them with the fighting Boomer Power than comes from getting with the life-empowering Boomer Smarts. Why would we want any less for ourselves, why wouldn't we want to be our best Boomer for all those we love and care about in our individual circles?

Remember, dear Boomer, every single choice you make definitely affects those in your personal or professional circle. For example, if you get enough sleep in your lifestyle routine, you are totally a different person than when you do not. In all areas of wholeness, like controlling stress, eating right, getting exercise, etc., living the life of Boomer Power in daily routines not only gives the best to our life but to all those we care so deeply about because even Boomers cannot give away what they themselves do not have. It is a law of nature, and even Boomers can't break that law and get away with it, either to themselves or to those they love and care about.

I absolutely believe in the thousands of my fellow Boomers who will indeed fight this battle of aging in America. They will do so with such gusto that all will know and see the results of their empowering lifestyle routines giving them the life other Boomers only envy from afar because those Boomers did not choose to equip themselves with the Boomer Smarts that enable lives to experience the ultimate Boomer Power.

So to the Boomer on the sideline of life, start fighting and fight hard to be all you were meant to be in your health with renewed energy and a zest for seizing new adventures and opportunities that are waiting for you to experience. I believe you can do it, and if you believe this too, watch out, your world will never be the same. You'll see.

Healthy Cooking and Eating Routines

Two beautiful and healthy-looking ladies I know personally had heart issues recently. Both live in the Dallas area, one is in her forties and was diagnosed with congestive heart failure and the other is in her sixties and had a serious heart attack.

Wow! Talk about a life-changing "are you kidding me?" Neither woman was overweight, neither woman smoked, and both are at their prime with their familiies and careers and yet, wham! Did I mention that they were beautiful and not overweight and yet still…

I have often said and written that life indeed can change on a dime, or in other words, one health issue or one whatever…

And yet, we do have control on how we do our part to give ourselves our very best odds to prevent chronic disease, and my Boomer Smart Boomers are all on board to do just that very thing—become proactive in their lifestyle routines! Later in this chapter, we will cover all of what a healthy lifestyle routine involves, including, of course, stress release, exercise, etc.

We all know that a huge part of this lifestyle routine is healthy eating and cooking. Statistics indicate 244,000 women die annually of heart disease, and 44,000 women die annually of breast cancer. Shouldn't that move us to live a lifestyle that gives us our very best odds right now?

But, of course, I know that life happens to the most healthy amongst us, but what is most disturbing is to hear over and over such negative talk:

"I am going to eat what I want and when I want. At my age, I have tons of time to figure it out." Oh really?

"This is just the way I have always been eating and looking; I enjoy my life eating my fast food, soda, cookies, and whatever else I have always done, and I am doing just fine the way I am." Oh really?

There is no more debate as to whether lifestyle and diet affect heart disease, cancer, arthritis, and diabetes. This is why it saddens me to see so many of my fellow Boomers totally disregarding their lifestyle choices.

But to the Boomers Who Are Learning and Doing Boomer Smart Lifestyle Routines, Their Rewards of Healthy Living Will Be Way Beyond the Typical American Baby Boomer.

You'll see.

What Boomer Smart Eating and Cooking Looks Like

Well, in my Boomer Smart lifestyle routine, there are no diet meals!

Boomer Smart eating and cooking is about healthy eating choices and healthy cooking, which will be shared in this section. Finding what eating plan, whether it is the Mediterranean way of eating or any of the other healthy plans, is the key to getting and maintaining Boomer Smart health. Extreme plans rarely work in the long run, and most people gain their weight back as soon as they begin eating "normal" again. Save yourself heartache, discouragement, and frustration and go for the long-term benefit of eating and cooking healthy...period.

And I use lots and lots of Boomer Smart meals that use "secret" tricks to fool the palate and the tummy that my food is actually healthy just because it tastes sooooo fabulous!

On my blog www.MitziBeach.com, there are many posts and videos on cooking healthy, fast, and delicious. Also, on my Pinterest boards are tons of recipes for all kinds of tastes and occasions, which are still healthy and mostly fast and always yummy. After all, add enough cheese, salt, fried anything, sour cream, and all that stuff and what wouldn't taste good??

So check the blog out for exact recipes and suggestions. Our purpose here is to share my theory of cooking and eating the Boomer Smart way that will equip you to incorporate these principles into any recipe (almost) or any way of eating and cooking.

So here we go, my really Smart Boomers...

I have had a love affair with food for as long as I can remember. In my family, we ate real food. Home cooked. We hardly ever ate anything packaged, and I can still see my dad going down the street to get clean fresh water out of a lovely, pure spring surrounded by thick velvety luscious green moss.

I am a foodie. I live to eat not eat to live. If it is not good food, I'm not eating it just to eat, and I make no apologies for that! I think about my meals every day, and most days I honestly and truly have a plan. And yes, even if it is just for me. Most people cannot even believe this is my daily routine. But this is how I maintain my weight and my precious health that I hold so dearly, never taking it for granted.

You are probably wondering why an interior designer would be so passionate about food, nutrition, and cooking, and truthfully, I do not have an answer other than design is design in all of life, and creativity is in designing meals as well as interiors.

I look at and actually visually savor the awesomely beautiful colors of food. I always say, how can anything improve on nature's palette? To put sweet potatoes, broccoli, and a perfectly cooked grain-fed beef filet on my plate is like an artist's composition in my eyes.

Way back, and I mean way back, I graduated from Ohio University with a degree in home economics education. Their program was unexpectedly challenging, with most of my professors having written their textbooks; they took no prisoners on their students' performance. For food science, chemistry was part of the curriculum for learning about microorganisms—not what I thought I was getting into for sure.

At any rate, it was the perfect background for really learning nutrition and all about food. It is still with me today, moving especially into another stage of life where diet needs change and, therefore, so should our food we eat…or do not eat.

So for me to finally have the opportunity to actually design my own kitchen, as I wrote in chapter one on spaces, was a life-long dream come true because, as I've expressed, I actually do cook. I considered carefully what would work for me appliance-wise to do my cooking. And seven years later of living at Cypress, I am still thrilled with my decision to include a built-into-the-counter steamer.

A steamer is such a healthy way to cook, and it is fast and also delicious. I do chicken, seafood, and veggies, always experimenting with different liquids such as orange juice, wines, chicken broth, even beer, along with good ol' water. I have looked and looked, however, and have found very little on steam cooking so far, other than what comes with appliances. Maybe someday I will do a Boomer Smart steam cooking cookbook. Ha! I can hear my sister, Kim, laughing all the way from Ohio at this idea! When, is the question, of course, but still...

I do virtually no cooking in the microwave that we have upstairs at Cypress. There is one included in our Thermador Smart Oven in our main kitchen, but it bears no relation to Boomer Smarts, however! I believe the food experts who say microwaves destroy the enzymes in fruit and vegetables; I do not microwave our veggies. I know, I know, sounds un-American! But, wisdom from science tells us that if our own digestive enzymes change and

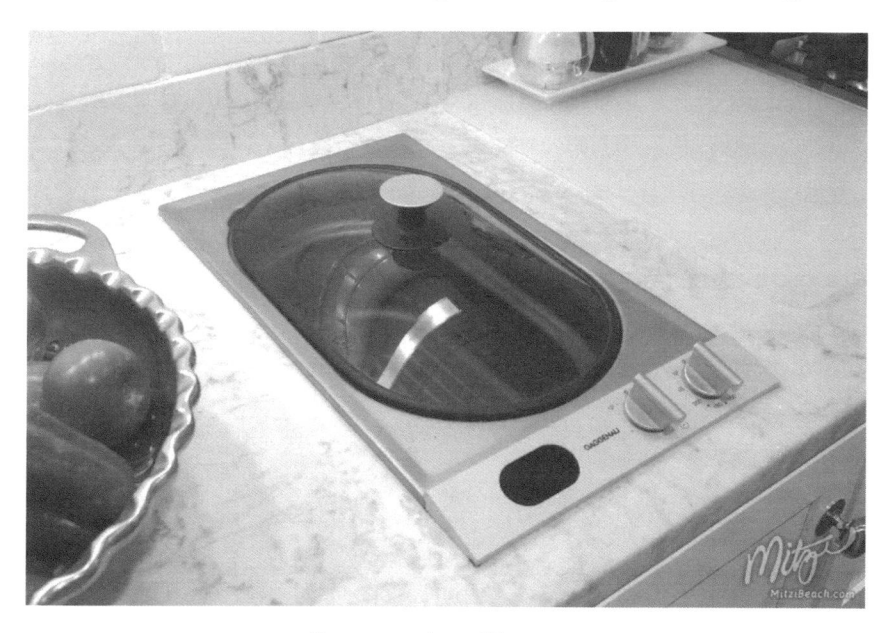

In-counter Steamer.

our bodies change as we age, don't we need all the nutrients we can possibly get out of our foods?

What's for Dinner?

Oh, man, how that simple question can so haunt us with pressure, frustration, guilt, and a zillion other feelings... seriously and really, right?

I in no way want to add more pressure, frustration, guilt, or a zillion other feelings when suggesting or showing Boomer Smarts examples of how to do it smarter and easier and also, I might add, healthier and cheaper.

There are 78 million Baby Boomers born between 1946 and 1964, and most are too tired or too busy to cook... seriously and really, right?

I hear it *all* the time from Boomers, and the most common of all these verbal statements is "it's only me" or "it's only me and my husband," so why bother with cooking?

A close second is, "Are you actually serious about cooking dinner? With our crazy schedules?"

I know, I know! My schedule is really crazy, too, on lots of days, but...

The answer to those comments is YES, it is important to learn Boomer Smart Cooking, which is:

1. HEALTHY

2. FAST

3. DELICIOUS

So who wouldn't like or want to cook like this instead of grabbing fast food and eating on the run all the time?

Whether we want to admit it or not, when we are tired, stressed, and overwhelmed with daily life, knowing what to cook is our biggest obstacle. It is not that we do not want to be and to eat healthier, but so much of the time it is the, "What in tarnation am I going to eat now because I am exhausted and I am starving here already!"

Do you know that it takes us eighteen attempts to learn a new habit? Well, learning Boomer Smart cooking is no exception, so it will not just happen by trying for a week and going back to those same ol' habits of grab and eat. Be kind to your Boomer self and give yourself a break; do not give up your attempts to learn a new habit.

Don't try to eat the elephant in one bite. We are so hard on ourselves that if we mess up, we often want to give up. Hang in there and keep on keeping on, even if it means only one time a week you don't grab and eat but cook at home a healthy, fast, and a delicious Boomer Smart meal. Then, the next week, cook two meals at home. There are a zillion sites out there on healthy cooking, zillions of books, and zillions of TV shows with all kinds of information—and yet, the dilemma remains. For the millions of overworked and overwhelmed Baby Boomers, on any given night, there are cries of, "What's for dinner???" A haunting reality of Boomer life today.

Why is it so hard to eat and cook healthy, especially when we know about the downfall of eating out routinely versus only occasionally?

I totally believe we have lost our way of finding and achieving the ultimate Boomer health simply because everyone else is doing the exact same thing. Right? We feel so justified and so less guilty when we hear others agreeing with what we do, whether it is healthy or not, because everyone else is doing it, too!

But again, the very big but here is that our bodies have not and will not adapt to our "new normal" way of eating out or bringing home fast or convenient food all the time. We simply cannot change the way our bodies were designed to function. Especially essential in Boomer aging is not lessening our healthy habits—kicking them up a notch is a must.

Why?

We all deserve to be healthy and not only just for ourselves. It's obvious, but perhaps not always realized, that our health directly affects in uncalculated ways those we love and care about in our personal Boomer lives.

So, how do we accomplish this new habit?

Keep It Simple, Sister (Or Brother)

It is amazingly easy to keep a few simple and very basic principles in our planning, buying, and cooking.

Step #1. Decide what lean protein you will have, such as chicken, lean beef, and fish, or if you are a vegetarian, what beans or grain you will have, such as quinoa.

Step #2. Add vegetables, whether in a salad, steamed, or stir-fried.

Step #3. If a carbohydrate is needed or wanted for certain dishes, do not choose an "all-white" carb, such as white flour, white rice, white pasta, white sugar, etc. Whole grains are the right choice the majority (perhaps eighty percent) of the time.

And speaking of eighty percent, again and again and again, I will reinforce my living healthy philosophy in all areas, and that is simply doing "my healthy thing" eighty percent of the time and my "not so healthy" only twenty percent of the time.

Translated, this means that most of the time I am doing the Boomer Smart eating method, but occasionally, by golly, I will have that pizza, chips and dip, ice cream, or whatever else my little Boomer craving wants and, by golly, I am going to savor and enjoy it to the max

Since this is not an actual Boomer Smart cookbook (although I will have one in the future), I want to certainly give you suggestions on how and where to find these simple, healthy, fast, and delicious ideas for Boomer Smart Cooking.

1. An exact example of a Boomer Smart meal is the tilapia dinner I cooked on KSN TV. The link is http://bit.ly/Hsj9VX and the recipe is at http://bit.ly/1bTmJSh
2. Our holiday cookbook free download link is http://bit.ly/1hIKYHD
3. My Pinterest boards are chock-full of ideas for Boomer Smart Cooking: http://pinterest.com/mitzibeach
4. You can find Boomer Smart Cooking on my blog site, www.MitziBeach.com
5. You can read my post Armed and Ready to Do Serious Battle to Those Bulges at http://bit.ly/HGcxmU

Now, equipped with this go-to knowledge, just remember, we are THE BOOMERS!

We will be the ones to age differently and age better in America!

And it will definitely start with learning Boomer Smart cooking, equipping ourselves with Boomer Power health to do and be all we are meant to be and all we deserve to be.

As my late dad said over and over, without our health we have nothing. It doesn't matter the size of our bank account, or the size of our home, or what car we drive. Ask anyone with health issues, and I bet my bottom dollar they will agree with what my dad used to say: "Without our health, we have nothing."

So guard your Boomer health with Boomer Smart eating and cooking.

This is defintely a choice we all make every day, every week, every month, and every years. We choose what and how we eat.

Choose life, choose health, choose Boomer Smart eating and cooking.

This choice will so affect and determine the quality of your future Boomer years. Choose Boomer Smart and watch the rewards happen because they surely will.

You'll see.

Boomer Smart Balance and Wholeness

Did you ever observe people around you who are almost fanatical in their exercise routines, and yet they eat so poorly? Or friends or family who brag about how little sleep they get, unlike the rest of us poor folks who admit to actually needing sleep and going to bed early? Do you ever hear experts explaining how bad stress is for us, and yet they are way, way overweight themselves?

Of course you have! It is everywhere, and just because you haven't discerned this in others, let me open your eyes, so to speak, to see—really see—how most Boomers are living their lifestyle routines. They have tunnel vision and often do not see the wholeness principle connected to Boomer Health.

Now, for sure, absolutely none of us accomplishes this wholeness and balance every day. That is like saying, "I am perfect and I do all things perfectly." PLEASE, spare me!

No, we are directing our focus to the everyday Boomer who is really trying to make a difference in their lifestyle routines, knowing and accepting the fact that life does indeed happen, and when it throws us off "balance," we do not berate or belittle ourselves. Again, we just recognize this unplanned detour and simply redirect ourselves when we can get back on track.

Our mission as Baby Boomers with Boomer Smarts is to live a life of Balance and Wholeness in all areas of life. These areas include:

Eating Habits
Exercise
"Social Toetherness"

Wholeness Living

Being a size eight or getting to the gym five days a week is not all there is to achieving wholeness. Let's dig deeper into this wholeness principle towards living in ultimate Boomer Power. But to really absorb and process these principles of Boomer Smarts for balance and wholeness, we must do the following as our catalyst to Boomer Power living.

Achieve Balance

Apply Knowledge

Prioritize You

These three principles are obviously obvious, right? We will learn the concepts of achieving balance next, but applying knowledge is, of course, clear. We must *apply* what we know or quit fooling our cute little Boomer selves.

And the third principle of *prioritizing you* is also very clear. Boomers cannot, as we have written and expounded on, simply cannot be all they are meant to be to themselves and others if they do not make themselves a priority! Who has the hardest time with this third principle?

Well, it is women, of course! They almost gasp thinking, "How selfish are you, Mitzi Beach, to put yourself first? Why, that is the most self-centered, egotistical thing I have ever heard." Oh, really?

Then tell me this, dear Boomer Woman, who will take care of those you love and those you have responsibility for if you are not able to do so? Who will pay for your health and medical needs if you are not up to your normal self needing health care? And how loving are you when you are so fatigued and overwhelmed from giving, giving, giving and never restoring the you in you?

So tell me again, who is being selfish? The Boomer Woman who takes care of herself or the Boomer Woman who ignores her own needs? Most women put their needs on the "if I have time" part of their life-strangling to-do lists, and I am no exception. This is an area where I really struggle, not because I do not value my own self-care, but I allow other things often to crowd out what I need and should be doing.

So, we will journey together on achieving this life of balance and wholeness through these lifelong goals. And, for sure, they are to be our Boomer lifelong goals, not a flash in the pan, short-term emotional decision. Oh, no, most certainly not; these goals are for our beautiful journey into the ultimate Boomer-Powered living.

Balance in Mind, Body, and Spirit

As I was determining how and what areas to include when writing this book, and what to address for obtaining a Boomer Smart life, going back to the basics was the only authentic answer for what to share, as I believe that all three—mind, body, and spirit—are part of who we all are. So, as we are looking at all the areas of Boomer Smarts—Spaces, Mindsets, Attitudes, Routines,

Togetherness, and Spirituality—not to reinforce how all the areas of mind, body, and spirit are included in the S.M.A.R.T.S. acronym could be incomplete and inconclusive without reinforcing the repetition that all of these categories are totally essential in my beliefs on how to live the Boomer-Powered life.

The Boomer Smart Formula for the
Best Rest of Life Eating Habits

We all know what we should be doing to eat healthy, but here are a few more suggestions. What works for me is basically eating clean foods, which really are just plain old good for us—nothing processed, little or no fast food, low salt, no bad fats, and organic when possible. But, remember, I am a foodie, so delicious and healthy are clearly not an oxymoron.

Eating habits greatly affect our weight, and controlling those pounds is essential in obtaining a life of Wholeness and Balance. We simply cannot be in Balance being thirty to fifty pounds over what our good weight is, and, of course, all Boomers already know this fact; the challenge is in the doing, to apply the knowledge. Isn't that truly all of life? Since we have covered Boomer Smart cooking and eating already, we will move on to...

Exercise

Get moving! I heard a truly disturbing statistic recently that retirees watch six to eight hours of TV a day! That is a "holy cow" thought for sure! If some Boomers are retiring in their mid-fifties and live to their mid-eighties, that's a whole lotta wasted time, in this Boomer's opinion. This includes watching sports, weather, news, and the like, but still, how much of life is being compromised by this one fact alone? More about this life-draining routine in the Togetherness chapter, but this must be acknowledged here in covering exercise as a critical component to living our best rest of our lives.

The type of exercise is as important as exercising itself. Weight-bearing exercise for bone health, aerobic exercise for heart health, and yoga, Pilates, or the like for our physical balance—all are necessary to achieve the optimum Boomer life of health and wholeness.

I personally love walking outside, which is my weight-bearing routine, and most walks are aerobic. I also love yoga for stretching and balance. But here, also, I simply need to do more of both, which is my intention. We all know what road is paved with good intentions, right?

Maintaining our body posture is a biggie, and doing exercise makes us more and more aware of our posture—another area I have to keep working hard on. As we age, it is so easy to slouch instead of forcing our muscles to work by putting those shoulders back, lifting our head up, and tucking that ol' tummy in. Be proud of who you are and how you look. It will definitely make a difference in your self-esteem. Try it and you'll see for yourself.

Besides the gym or a personal trainer, there are so many options to us for exercise. Swimming, walking, biking, or exercise DVDs work wonders. I love my yoga DVD from our famous Flora Edwards, a Wichita, Kansas, icon well in her eighties and still going strong—literally. Find something you love. Or maybe that is too strong an emotion for some of you Boomers regarding your exercise. Perhaps find something you at least enjoy!

Balanced Living

Of all the areas to wholeness, living a balanced life is what I hear most Boomers lamenting on how to do. With so many demands today on lives that seem to be busier than ever, how do we really ever achieve the ultimate balance in life?

I only know that I would be lying out my teeth if I professed to leading a balanced life. Here again, I am doing tons better, but I have a long way to go on these areas of achieving balance, which are:

Adequate Sleep

Another biggie for sure, as a sleep study by the Center for Disease Control indicates that thirty percent of the US working population, or about 40 million Americans, get less than six hours of sleep a night. Another poll by the National Sleep Foundation indicated forty-five percent get less than seven hours of sleep each night. That's more than just a lot of sleepy people, as inadequate sleep robs us of our immunity and our health!

Adequate sleep results in:

Fewer aches and pains
Better moods and emotional stamina
Sharper thinking and ability to focus
Easier to maintain weight control
Increase in memory recall

Sleep is not just a luxury for when we have the time, but a serious need in our quest for better health, not to mention our quality of life. We know now that a good night's sleep is a big factor in our longevity, which makes perfect sense if we look at the above lists.

Controlling Stress

Oh my, I have written many blog posts on this subject,

and there is no end in sight of what we are learning on the negative and life-draining effects of stress. One of the most significant advances in our medical pursuit of the whys of disease is...you guessed it correctly if you said stress. And one of the main underlying culprits of stress in our lives is that it physically causes inflammation. Many medical professionals believe the inflammation that stress causes is directly linked to heart disease, diabetes, cancer, arthritis, and other serious and chronic diseases.

When stress-induced inflammation occurs in our bodies, our cortisol levels increase, which is not a good thing. What was once commonly called the flight or fight syndrome, an increase in adrenalin for our bodies to kick into high gear in times of real danger or real crisis, is now how many people live on a day-to-day basis. Just plain-old common sense tells us that eventually we are going to wear ourselves out living in this state or pattern.

But in today's crazy world, it is not only assumed that we are going to be on call 24-7, it is expected!

This is where I throw in the towel. I am not a machine. I do not and will not be available 24-7 for whoever feels their needs are so important that I am negligent if I do not respond on their timetable. This is a huge Boomer step for me, and especially one for a recovering people pleaser. I will give my all during my defined working hours, giving and being all that I possibly can to contribute, influence, or assist others. But when my day is over, it is over. And you know what? I am not the least bit guilty about it!

Of course life issues happen, and of course for a very few key people and my precious family and grandchildren, I am open 24-7. But that is as far as I am willing to sacrifice my health in maintaining my balance of shutting down and turning off and tuning out.

Routines

But correcting our Boomer lifestyle routine is soooo much more difficult than taking a pill, right? You see, we are still in the mindset that getting high blood pressure medicine or meds for the type 2 diabetes or arthritis or other issues is the only answer. Our "take a pill" mindset allows us to continue to function as we always have, and is for the most part our medical way of life or our path to health in America today.

I do not believe this is the way it has to be, and I do not live my own life this way. My first line of defense is "what can I do differently to avoid all these medical ailments, and if they occur, what life change can I make to avoid taking meds?" This is all part of the formula for being proactive in seeking our Boomer Balance and Wholeness.

Balance and Wholeness are, assuredly, the Boomer key to unlock those doors to walking in the ultimate Boomer Power of living a healthy life.

Just even thinking of the word "wholeness" gives the impression of nothing missing, nothing broken. Only with sincere introspection into our Boomer lives will the out-of-balance areas be revealed. Take the time to discern and process if your life is lacking in balance like your life depends on it. Go through the Boomer Wellness Meter below. Yes, my dear fellow Boomer, wholeness is possible. You'll see.

Boomer Smart Wellness Meter

Boomer Smart wellness is all about wholeness...not perfection. It is about being healthy and not about being a size eight or getting to the gym five days a week. Oh no, it is so much more involved for optimum wholeness and wellness in achieving the ultimate Boomer life with a Boomer Power lifestyle.

Obtaining Boomer Smart wholeness includes:

Healthy Eating Habits or Routines
Having a Balanced Life
Exercise Routine
Social "Togetherness"

And the not-so-scientific but so-revealing tool for balance and wholeness is our

Boomer Smart Wellness Meter

In this Boomer Smart Wellness Meter, there is no total scoring or graphs, just a simple *N* for not so good, a *G* for good, and a *B* for best. No one sees how whole or balanced the Boomer checking their meter is.

Perhaps someday we will have a measuring scale, but for now, just our own knowledge is worth EVERYTHING in our quest to seek and realize balance and wholeness in our Boomer lives.

Rate each of the following as:

N for Not so good / hardly ever,

G for Good / most days,

B for Best / 80% of the time

Eating Habits

_____ Eat three meals daily
_____ Eat colorful fresh fruits and veggies (most diets are earth tones or neutral in color)
_____ Avoid fast food
_____ Cook at home or buy healthy, already-prepared food to take home
_____ Eat leans protein or grains high in protein, such as quinoa
_____ Have low-sugar foods and drinks
_____ Have low-salt foods, avoid processed foods high in salt
_____ Read labels for hidden sugars, salt, high-fructose corn syrup, etc.
_____ Have no or little soda
_____ Eat healthy snacks
_____ "Police weight" regularly
_____ Drink lots of water daily

Exercise

_____ Weight-bearing exercise, such as walking, to maintain bone strength and bone health; lifting weights
_____ Aerobic exercise that gets the heart rate up, such as swimming
_____ Exercising at least three or four times weekly, incorporating weight-bearing and aerobic-type exercises
_____ Stretching exercising, such as yoga or Pilates
_____ Exercise for improved balance
_____ Work on posture

Having a Balanced Life

_____ Time alone for unwinding

_____ Get seven to eight hours of sleep a night
_____ Control stress by whatever mentally or emotionally detoxifies
_____ Learn to recognize the "crazies" in life and how to deal or not deal with them
_____ Take time just for yourself without feeling guilty
_____ Take mental health days off
_____ Find something that gives you joy and doing it
_____ Find your passion or hobby
_____ Value yourself enough to schedule time for what needs you have, such as a massage
_____ Spend time with those you love, such as family or friends
_____ Stay connected socially
_____ Allow for free time during the day, not scheduling yourself so tightly

Social "Togetherness"

_____ Make time for family
_____ Make time for friends
_____ Schedule time to connect with others
_____ Find meaningful causes or groups to become involved with or to contribute your time and expertise
_____ Get out of your too-tight schedule and connect with someone
_____ Get out of yourself and your to-do lists

There it is, the original Boomer Smart Wellness Meter.
Where or how would you rate yourself?
What areas need improvement?
What are your specific personal improvement plans toward Boomer Wholeness?
Remember, dear fellow Boomer, life is made up of choices. What you choose to do or incorporate today will

Routines

absolutely affect what or how you look and feel five years from now.

Go for it! Live and enjoy your Boomer life that you were meant to have and live. If you do, the best is yet to come. You'll see.

Boomer Smart Stories

Mary Baldwin

Mitzi: It's been really, really exciting having these interviews with mover and shaker women like yourself, Mary. And actually, except for you in Kansas City and Cindy Carnahan here in Wichita, all the others I have met or have been connected with are through social media or from attending conferences with women all over the country.

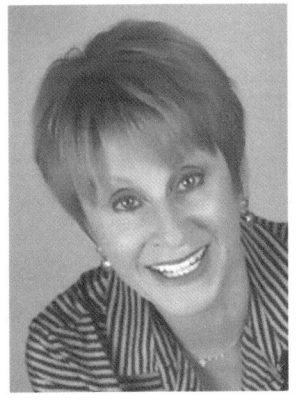

It's been really affirming how many women are trying to just get through life and are struggling with a lot of the same questions. And many Boomers are not exactly struggling but are pondering and thinking out of the box now that aging questions are in front of them or until it's brought up.

And so, they were very encouraging to me about moving forward and really digging in to this whole arena of what our future looks like and the health; of course, you and I had been passionate about it for a long time. But we're the—what's the word? The minority, don't you think? Kansas City probably isn't as typical as maybe Wichita and other areas, that all we have to do is look at the airport or go somewhere and it's just like, oh—your heart aches for them. "Oh, man, if they only knew about what is ahead for them if they don't start paying attention to themselves."

You know, it's where most Americans I think are in a naïve bubble. They just have no clue what lies ahead for them. So, we're hoping to shake them up on that. And so, I know you're part of this physical, the health part of this chapter is not because you have been all along neglecting your health, but just the opposite.

So, the first question for you is, Mary, that your most significant health life was your breast cancer ordeal, but I don't want to assume. Am I correct on that, or is there some other—

Mary: Well, there are others, two of them.

Mitzi: Okay. And so, how does that alter your future, your health future, besides what happens?

Mary: It was just an absolute commitment, a personal commitment on my part to stay strong and as strong—physically strong—and fit as I see throughout the rest of my life.

Mitzi: Was the issue shocking to you? I mean, when you found out that the test...were you blown out of the water, so to speak, or because of your family history, how does that diagnosis or that test result...?

Mary: Okay, the diagnosis of my potential breast cancer, of course that scared me to death, but I also had taken my health for granted. And so, that was such an eye opener for me, and I chose to have this mastectomy, and because I was not going to have that fear factor of, you know, am I going to deal with this breast cancer in the future because I did have a family history of it with my mother. So I didn't even have to think about it. I knew that I was going to have the surgery within five minutes after the doctor told me I had some potential for cells, cancer cells in the future.

Mitzi: What determined that? Was it blood work, or did

you have a lump, or how was that...?

Mary: They found it in a routine mammogram. And—how am I going to say it...? I just feel so thankful for that technician when she saw something—and she could have passed it by because it was so small—and she doublechecked it.

Mitzi: Oh, my goodness—

Mary: She sent me to a breast specialist and they just went, "Oh, you know, really, we don't have to do anything, but if we don't, you know, this could catch on fire, you know, in the next year or so, and so I just sat there that day, and I had just been through breast cancer with my sister-in-law, and she was with me that day, and I just went, "You know, I'm not doing this." That's when I just decided that day I was going to have the surgery. But because of my good health and my exercise through the years up to that point, I absolutely know that was what got me through that surgery and my recovery, because I was strong in that.

Mitzi: Excellent. Excellent way to be encouraging other women. I haven't considered that side of it, but we all know that being in tip-top shape to prepare fighting for whatever could raise its ugly head is important. I haven't thought about it, Mary, from the angle of those of us that are not dealing with anything currently; it doesn't give us a free pass to not be in the best physical health.

Mary: Correct, correct.

Mitzi: Right? It's what you discovered. I mean, had you

been forty pounds overweight and had not been exercising and whatnot, it truly would have been…I mean, not that it's a walk in the park, your recovery, but it could have been a lot different.

Mary: Very much so. So, I'm just—I absolutely believe that even if you are fit and healthy, it is felt in your after care, and you'll recover it.

Mitzi: Awesome. I'm even hearing—well, there's a program now, "something forward." I don't think it's pay it forward, that phrase, but programs are here for those scheduled for knee and hip replacements to get into an exercise and health care routine before their procedures.

And it cuts the…And one of the reasons that we're talking about being in good physical condition is so many women, and we've all been there and we have seasons when it doesn't occur, but we put ourselves last and we don't make the time, right, to focus on ourselves, and do what we need to do. And I think that's a woman's Achilles' heel. You're not on that mindset, Mary, but I'm sure you know people that—

Mary: Oh, but I think I am. I think every woman is of that mindset in varying degrees. That, you know, I have—I just have made that commitment and you know, Pilates is my choice.

Mitzi: And it shows.

Mary: But I just think Pilates or yoga is an absolute must for Baby Boomer women.

Mitzi: Good point.

Mary: But in my Pilates studio, I am the oldest one there, and I look around and go, "Where are all these women my age that should be here?" I don't understand that.

Mitzi: Excellent point, Mary. Excellent.

Mary: I don't understand that. It's all the young chicks, and it's the Baby Boomers in their fifties, sixties, and seventies that need to be there.

Mitzi: Oh, you're right. But do you see why they need to be there, Mary, for the Pilates, for how it helped you?

Mary: For the strength and for the flexibility and I think…And that is true with yoga. And I think cardio is important, but I think yoga or Pilates is the utmost number one priority.

Mitzi: Good, good advice.

Mary: Being flexible and strong, it helps with all of life. Whether it's picking up groceries out of your car, picking up a grandbaby that's running towards you, you know. I mean that's a total joy to be able to lean down and pick up a baby, and you know, it's just for the practical sense of moving about every day and—

Mitzi: Just what we take for granted, and if we're not in core condition or flex condition, to pull our back out in a nanosecond doing something insignificant because the strength and flexibility are not there.

Mary: Absolutely, which brings me to my second issue, other than my surgery, was—

Mitzi: Okay.

Mary: ...my cute little mommy that has severe osteoporosis and from probably seventy on, and she was eighty-one when she died, but she was bent at a ninety-degree angle.

Mitzi: Oh my...

Mary: And I'll never forget when we had her in at an osteoporosis specialist in Kansas City, and they said, "Okay, you have a choice here. You can either exercise or you're going to be in a wheelchair for the rest of your life." And sadly, she decided—she ended up in a wheelchair instead of strengthening, and that really, really scared me.

So, I had two scares...two things, and I just firmly believe that things could have been different for her, and so that's why my exercise is preventative for me, and then I will admit it's vanity, too.

Mitzi: Yeah, me too.

Mary: Not as important at my age, but it's still there and I think you don't have anything else to lose by trying...not obsessing, but not giving up, either.

Mitzi: And I'm so glad you brought that up, Mary. It's okay for us to care about what we look like, and I haven't even considered, anticipated doing that part of physical care. But it is extremely important to a Boomer's self-esteem and self-confidence no matter what some say with the "I don't give a damn, Scarlett" attitude.

And not only for how we feel but for the role model

that we give to those around us, right?

Mary: Absolutely, and I also see other family members of mine that could have benefited from exercise and nutrition but chose not to go that direction.

Mitzi: Uh huh, I know, and it's a fine line, isn't it? Especially with family.

Mary: Uh huh.

Mitzi: What there is to say, and really, most of the time we can't say. So, it's like so many other things, and you and I, I know, agree on this, that we show about what we do and just be that example. And you are such a fabulous example, Mary. It's one of the reasons I wanted to have you involved, in that Boomer women need Boomer role models.

And I spent two chapters in this book on opening up Boomer minds. One is our mindsets, which can be called strongholds, whether it's positive or negative. But I'm talking about the negative, and the paradigm of the aging of acceptance. And then another chapter on attitude, and of course, they play into the health in the home because if we're not…if we don't have a teachable spirit, if we're not willing to learn, and if we're not willing to put our pride aside and listen to whatever people perhaps can glean from us, no matter what anybody writes, it's simply going to be ignored.

So, that's why I have the interviews in the book, to indeed show other women that not only read the book but hear about what other Boomers are thinking and doing. Of course, most importantly is that we don't have to be this way. There's a better way, and not that I have all the answers, but these are some of the things that will be a help to these Boomers. And the top goal is to get Boomers out of this; I called it the herd mentality, where you hear Boomers say, "Oh, I have all my friends look like this," or, "Everyone is on high blood pressure medicine," or, "What? You're not taking a statin?" And no—we're not accepting that, are we? I mean, we don't want to and we don't. We know we don't have to, but unless we stick out of the crowd, and even if it's just by our look, how we act, what we're able to do, hopefully, others will want that too. And you know, if we would reach twenty people, hallelujah!

Mary: Hallelujah!

Mitzi: Okay. So, three, what has been the result of your decisions? And of course, you said peace of mind, but the result, Mary, not—there's been a lot of women that have had a mastectomy and breast replacement.
 The emotional part of having a mastectomy, did you have any issues with that or were you so focused on healing and moving forward? If some women have said they grieved losing their breasts, you know, I have no way of relating to that because I've never been there.

Mary: Ask me.

Mitzi: Some are grieving about losing their breasts when they have to have a mastectomy. It's not like women that are going in for implants. They're doing these for preventative reasons. And did you have any second thoughts about the way your body looked or anything like that, that part of it?

Mary: You know, that's interesting, I didn't. I do remember standing in the mirror before the implants were in, and then the nipple reconstruction, and you can say whatever you want to say. You can take that however you want. And I really—after a period of time, after a couple of months, I just couldn't look at myself anymore. I wanted to look normal. And so, that's when I just went on, what's the next steps, and did the implant and the whole reconstruction procedure. But I guess that was a sense of grieving. That's difficult for me to answer because I don't remember. I was just so relieved, so relieved not to have that potential there anymore.

Mitzi: Plus, I think you also had prepared yourself. You said that you were allowing yourself months to…when you were going to try to get back to what you thought would be normal. Anyways, in your mind, Mary, you were calculating that this was going to be the time of healing, and that's what it's going to be.

So, maybe because you were already determined you were going to have to go through whatever it was. It was not known but you knew by your words to—I heard you say that you had to go through to get to the other side. And how did you know what that looked like? But I so admired that thinking, that you had prepared yourself emotionally besides the health part, you know, just being—

Mary: Well, and I think I did, Mitzi, and just going through that with my sister-in-law or with family with her radiation and her chemo with breast cancer, I think it was more relief that I wasn't going to have to do any of that. It overpowered the sense of loss of my breasts.

Mitzi: Oh. Okay. Because you have seen firsthand how devastating and—

Routines

Mary: Yeah. It was worth it to me. Okay, go ahead.

Mitzi: The last question is, of course, one that you probably can have a long, quickie answer, and I don't expect that, but what tip or advice would you give to other Boomer women regarding their health issues and their health futures?

Mary: Well, of course I think my big focus is on staying strong and flexible. And women, they have to get over feeling guilty about taking that time. It does take time to go to a Pilates class or even exercising at home, but you have to commit to that time and absolutely work your life scheduling around it because it's the number-one priority. And it's not to feel self-indulgent.

Mitzi: Uh huh.

Mary: I mean, I think a lot of women, you know, feel selfish just not taking time for themselves to get and be healthy. Time to go to classes, and then they also—and I do not abide by this at all, where they say, "I don't have time."

Mitzi: I know.

Mary: Well, I think that is a foolish thing.

Mitzi: Excellent. And what about food and eating? I hear so much about our life stage, when there are so many single women now that say—and I'm talking our age single; somebody told me today, this lady from New York, that approximately seventy percent of women were single, and I was shocked at that. I told her I'd heard fifty percent.

Mary: Really?

Mitzi: I don't remember the statistic or the percentage, but it is way, way reversing from families to singles, a lot, lot, a lot is happening with single people.

And so, the single women as well as us that are married, that are at this life stage, I can't tell you how many times I hear, "Well, it's just the two of us. I'm not going to cook," or "It's just me."

Mary: Right.

Mitzi: "Why would I..." So, what is your take on that, Mary? How do you take care of your health besides the physical part? And I don't mean to put you on the spot, even if you're not—

Mary: I eat well...nutritionally.

Mitzi: Okay. So, you do make that a priority also?

Mary: Absolutely, and you know, also, and I think which is pretty typical, was most people I mean, I— you and I have talked about this a lot, but where, you know, when I go up five or six pounds and I go even more healthy and try to get back to my reasonable weight. And I just think everybody has to do that almost on a quarterly basis, or things—quarterly to me because I'm just not going to carry that extra weight around my middle because of balance and core strengths.

Mitzi: Uh huh, okay. And as far as you and Gene and taking care of your nutrition or your eating or your food, do you fight the going out for the fast food? Do you have a pattern that you follow? How do you work that?

Mary: When we are at home, we eat healthy. We usually would have protein and vegetables. But we're probably fifty-fifty, fifty percent going out for dinner, fifty percent eating at home.

But I'm—it goes back to Mitzi Beach's formula of eighty-twenty, that's what I go by. And so, you know, I don't diet, I just eat fresh, even when I go out for dinner.

Mitzi: Okay. And so, what I'm hearing and what we can share is that even eating out, it doesn't necessarily take eating unhealthy to an unhealthy level?

Mary: Correct.

Mitzi: And I think we have to get over that black and white thinking that, "Oh, my gosh, what is, you know, I'm going out to eat. But there's nothing here...I'll have the side chips or whatever it may be." And that just is not true.

Mary: No, it really is not true.

Mitzi: And even to where we go to eat. It's very challenging to eat healthy in a Mexican restaurant. But you can do it—

Mary: Yes, you can. Uh huh. I think you have to pick and choose your restaurants, too. I mean, I haven't been in the fast food restaurant for ten years, other than getting coffee at McDonald's. You just can't do that. So—

Mitzi: It's not pretty. So, last question, and it's not really what I have intended to ask you, that as far as looking at your future, Mary, what would be the main thing that you're cognizant of? I mean what…what is out there for you that at all cost you're going to work against happening? Is it your history of osteo? Or don't you think about it?

Mary: It is the history of the osteo. That would be first and foremost for me. You know, stay strong and act right and then, also, my latest thing is exercising my brain power. And I don't know how to put that, but at sixty-four, I just—it's just—it's just first and foremost but I'm just working on it.

Mitzi: Good point, Mary. And there are so many studies also that are telling us that being physically fit is a direct correlation to our brain health and our mental capabilities. And you know, we can say that God is just so smart, how all of what we do is integrated. There isn't one part separate from the other. If you exercise, eat right, mental health—they're all part of how He designed us.

Mary: Exactly. And I guess, Mitzi, the challenge for me, as it is for most women, is balance. I don't think of balance, and then I have to check all of the time.

Mitzi: Yes, yeah. Oh, but that's very good. That's part of it because wholeness is about balance, and we can't have the Boomer Smart, Boomer Power—we can't be empowered without being in balance. If we're stressed to death, literally, if we're not exercising and if we're not—I mean, it's all the wholeness package. Mary, that was an excellent point. And it's the daily struggle for me. I mean daily—

Mary: Daily.

Mitzi: One of the ladies I've talked to—and she's single and has a career—she was talking about finding things for her that were fun because her life is so wrapped up in her career being her fulfillment and her whole life. She said exactly what you just said, but in another connotation. It was the balance to finding something else.

So, I think we're hearing a common trend of what all women struggle with, and that is the balance. And it's not like we have a formula and we can say, "Okay, this is what we're going to do, la la la la la," because every day is different and every family member is different every day, and life is different. And I think that—

Mary: Well, it's finding balance in everything that you are basing your book on. And it's just tough to do, but that's...that's our daily Baby Boomer challenge. Stay rested, eat well, exercise, you know. So—

Mitzi: Yeah. And the rewards are worth it!

Mary: Absolutely, absolutely.

Mitzi: We can't guarantee what life is going to bring. We have faith and we know that we're doing the best we can do, and that's all we can do. But we're going to do that to the best that we can because instead of having that comfy attitude of whatever will be, will be, no. We look, we're...we're going for it. So—

Mary: And Mitzi, I run into people that are my age that

I would like to, I just want to go up to them and say, "Stop, what are you doing? My goodness, when did you give up? When did you check it in?" You know? I see this so much, that you and I are around wonderful women most of the time, and you forget—

Mitzi: Right.

Mary: Earlier we said that there are so many that quit caring.

Mitzi: And I can see on Facebook, I can see when I visit women that I haven't seen in the family or friends, and it's like what you are thinking, Mary, "You gave up. I can see that you're giving in."

Mary: Right.

Mitzi: Do you know what I'm saying? And it's just they give up. So, I totally and I'm going to—I'm definitely writing that, and you know, again, the book is for those who have ears to hear and eyes to see and a mind to embrace. I'm not out to evangelize the world about this. There are people that are—and want to do—different, and that's the bottom line. And there are people, Mary, that we are never going to touch because they are very satisfied. They don't think anything differently, and sad, sad for them. I mean I just—I'm sad for them because it's not going to be pretty.

Mary: No, it's not. Yeah, it's not. But your book is so exciting, Mitzi, and I want to give it to so many people I love and care about in my life.

Chapter 5
Togetherness

Boomers with Boomer Smarts Live to Give

Loneliness Is a Choice: True or False?

The movers and shakers of the huge Baby Boomer generation are out there making waves and history again, but this time not by burning bras or protesting Viet Nam. No, they are doing amazing and unheard of pioneer-busting activities that literally are changing the world. It is called giving back, or another way to put it is that Boomers are getting out of themselves! Of course, we all have bouts with self-pity or depression or are just basically down in the pits sometimes, and not many Boomers are up 100% of the time and are not affected by life's up and downs.

But to be lonely can actually be a self-imposed condition. Now before you go stringing me up for writing this, think about what I actually mean. I am referring to the consequence of Boomers being self-centered or thinking and being obsessed with their own well being way more than thinking about how to help others.

Living with Purpose and Passion

Living a "it's not about me" life and getting out of ourselves into others' lives is a sure antidote for loneliness. A life with a purpose outside of ourselves is a life brimming over with satisfaction of doing something worthy for other people. Especially if helping others also falls outside of our immediate families. Now we're talking out of ourselves!

We can live in pity or purpose but not both at the same time.

Many Boomers, even those with chronic illness or who are compromised by accidents or myriad other conditions, have found ways to move beyond their afflictions to be involved in others' lives. Those Boomers who are giving back are statistically healthier and need less medical care and have fewer medical expenses. That's reason enough right there to give!

Boomers who give back have more friends, more fun, more new experiences, and more zest for life than those who stick to their own personal territory doing the same thing they have done their whole life with the same people they have known their whole life.

We value our friends and family, and they hold the highest priority in our lives most definitely. However, if the Boomer never moves beyond their network of family and friends to give of their time to myriad causes, to people outside their own circles, schools, churches, organizations, neighbors, hospitals, etc., not only are they missing out but so is their world being robbed of their talents, expertise, and experiences.

This is not rocket science—the loss of influence and potential for millions of Boomers to make a difference in America is real. My goodness, though, what does it take to get those millions of Boomers off their you-know-whats and get them out there doing the millions of things that need doing in our communities and in our country?

The "if you snooze you lose" saying is so very true for

Togetherness

Boomers. Just observe and witness these movers and shakers out there doing all kinds of innovative volunteering and starting of new programs...often while still working or starting another career and often while literally climbing a mountain somewhere or going on a lifelong dream trip to wherever. These Boomers are not snoozing their Boomer life away and in no way are losers in any sense.

The point is that getting out of ourselves and giving back does not mean Boomers do not get to do all the things we have wanted to do all our lives. And after prolonging our dreams and goals for families, paying college tuitions, paying for weddings, etc., of course Boomers are entitled to "their time."

Boomers with Boomer Smarts, however, understand without a doubt that the way to live the rest of their days in fulfillment is to give back up and beyond their own dreams and goals. This is a win-win not only for the Boomer, but for all those in their world they have given of their time, talents, and experience.

So loneliness for the Boomer with Boomer Smarts is just not a routine happening or a way of life. They are way too smart for that downer way of living. Oh no, remember, we are THE BABY BOOMERS, and we are still shaking up America by doing our thing in a totally different way than any other generation before us.

Fighting off the most feared and dreaded aspect of aging, loneliness, is just not part of how we intend to show who we are and how we Boomers age. You'll see.

Leaving a Legacy of Influence

No one told my mom, Ellen Garrett, that she could not possibly do all that she did way, way back in the forties, fifties, and up until the present.

She worked outside of the home as a telephone operator in the era of Donna Reed and Ozzie and Harriet, when moms stayed home. None of my friends' moms worked.

A funny thing that occurred in my very late adulthood was realizing the fact that we lived on the "other" side of town. Not for a second did this ever register to me, my position or my status, because my mom made life all very normal...like the other moms that never worked outside the home.

Even though she was working full time, it was always my mom who volunteered to be a Brownie and Girl Scout leader, who often made the cookies or brownies or brought food for us girls. I was a little girl that loved, loved her baby dolls, and my dolls had tons and tons of clothes made by, of course, my mom.

Then came junior and senior high and slumber parties! You guessed it...at my house in our basement. And, right again, she always made sloppy joes, brownies, chip and dip, etc., and let us stay up late, late, late, and never did I hear, "You girls be quiet, I have to work!"

Then I went away to college at Ohio University in Athens, Ohio, four *very* long hours away from my hometown. I still remember thinking how homesick I was. Small town girl at a university almost twice the size of my whole town's population.

So while Mom was still working full time, my mom and dad and sweet baby sister Kim traveled to Ohio U as much as their work would allow to visit me. And they were never empty handed on these family visits. Oh no, they were loaded down with, you guessed it...homemade brownies, chocolate chip cookies, fresh lilacs for my birthday month, and Villager knock-off dresses complete with matching headbands sewn, of course, by my mom.

No fast food then, no cleaning ladies, tons of ironing, my little sister still at home—and my mom and dad made

Togetherness

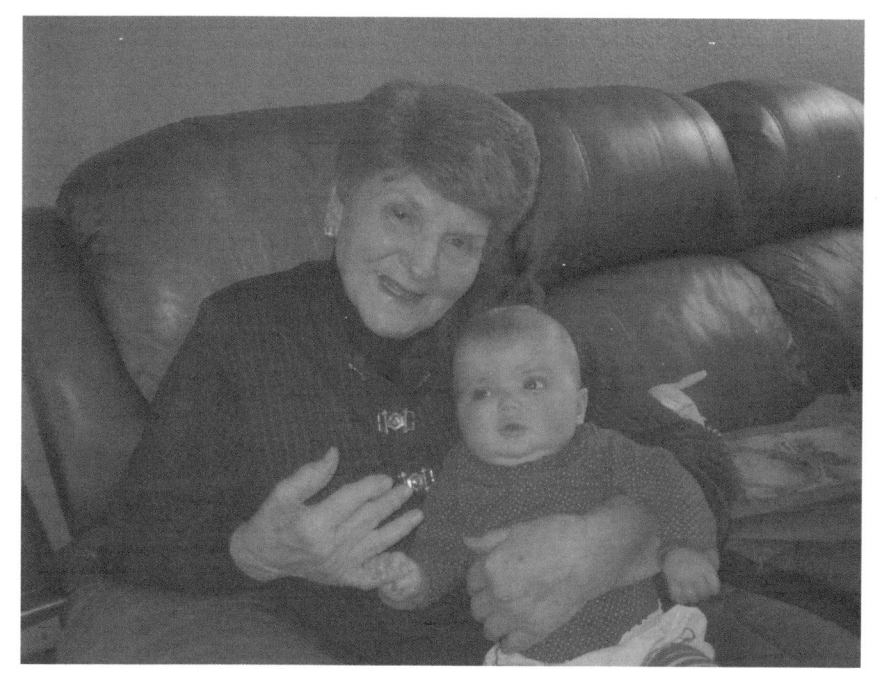

Ellen Garret Won't Let Anything Slow Her Down.

it all work. And work they did...very hard.

So look at Ellen Garret now in this photo, where she's pushing ninety, and know that she has not even slowed down to *her* age...she's maybe akin to someone in their seventies, perhaps.

She puts on her tennis shoes every Monday and for hours and hours she serves the needy in the Community Center in Salem, Ohio. Of course she is by far the oldest and confesses that she sneaks cookies to the little ones.

Up until very recently, you would have found her helping out at the food bank on Fridays, doing I'm sure whatever is asked of her.

And for many, many years, she and her friends have adopted a group of mentally disabled women, taking them on outings such as bowling, hot dog roasts in the park, movies, doing crafts, or taking them out to eat.

And, if I told you what homebaked food she packs in

suitcases to bring to our family, whether she's traveling by car or by plane, you probably would not believe it possible, but believe it. She even keeps a notebook of who likes what cookies and quantities and what to adjust for the next family get together...seriously!

Or, would you even believe me if I told you also that she still exercises and cooks *very* healthy meals for herself, even with my dad being gone now for years. She gets pretty feisty when she hears people say they won't cook because it is just themselves or just the two of them. Don't even get her started on that one. I love it!

I haven't even skimmed the surface of all that my mom is and all that she does for sooooooooo many people. And my dad, too, was always behind the scenes doing everything that needed to be done when it needed to be done for family and friends alike. Putting up shelves, delivering mom's cooking, washing, washing, washing, and washing tons of pots and pans! Yes, my dad would literally be the one giving "the shirt off his back," and tons of family friends' stories atest to this generous spirit of my dad too.

As I move into my future of launching Boomer Smarts to a new and different level, Ellen Garrett will always be in the back of my mind saying, "Who said you couldn't do this, Mitzi?" Because no one ever told her with any success that she could not accomplish all she did indeed do.

May I be half the woman that my mom is. She has shown her entire life that no matter what her circumstances, she is a woman of influence.

It is not about the applause, it is not about the numbers, it is not about recognition. No, the Boomers who leave a legacy of influence will have an impact on others that will extend way beyond their lifetime.

You'll see.

Togetherness

Boomer Smart Stories

Doreen Hanna
Modern Day Princess Ministry
www.ModernDayPrincess.net

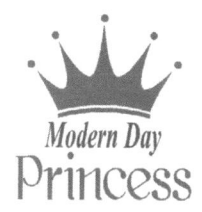

Modern Day
Princess

Mitzi: Please give us a glimpse or status of what your Modern Day Princess ministry looks like today.

Doreen: It's beyond my dream. So I'll just say that. I never thought that what I created in my mind as an American, Biblically based rite-of-passage would become an international need.

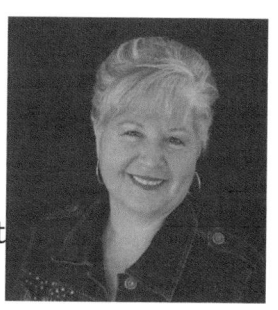

Mitzi: So Amazing, Doreen. Since you are one busy lady, let's get to why you are so important to include in my book, which I'm really excited about. It's to deal with us Boomers, and like your ministry, God put this in my heart years ago about preparing the Boomers for their future.

America is changing and changing quickly, and things that were, may or may not be available. So, the purpose of the book is to inspire, educate, and motivate Boomers to at least start considering their futures. And you know, a lot of people, and us included, are just scrambling as fast as we can, right? And so, trying to consider our future sometimes is something like whoa, I'm just trying to get through the day here.

But your chapter that I wanted to address is on Togetherness, which is about leaving a legacy, giving back, getting out of ourselves, thinking beyond the "my four and no more" mentality—this is where for millions of Boomers, their whole world is just right in front of their own family, and that's it. I'm not criticizing for a minute family as our priority, but there is so much potential in us Boomers, as you have shown.

So, my first question then is where were you in your Boomer life when the creating and developing of Modern Day Princesses happened? Were you at a crossroads? How did this happen at your Boomer stage?

Doreen: Okay. I was forty-nine, and I had been traveling with Women of Faith, and I was their first West Coast rep at that time. And during that period of time, it was coming to an end because they wanted me to move to their Plano, Texas, offices, and my husband had a very secure job at that time. And so, I knew that wasn't going to be an option. I was kind of on the B team for speakers for Women of Faith. So, that's how I got a call from a church in Torrance, California, here, asking me to come and speak on "Celebrate! You're a Daughter of the King" with the underlying message of the older women mentoring the younger women—and during that period of time, obviously, when I knew I wasn't going to continue with Women of Faith. And God puts this vision in my heart as I prepared this talk: that there isn't a Biblically based rite-of-passage for our American girls. I had seen big value of the Bob Smith material, or the Jewish community, and, of course, being in our culture here in California for the Hispanic community was very popular. So all of a sudden, God is placing this in my heart to develop the Modern Day Princess Program, which was basically a Biblically based rite-of-passage for our teen girls. And that being new on the market, I didn't know how that was going to go because our American culture didn't know what a rite-of-passage was.

Mitzi: No.

Doreen: So, that was a result of God prompting in my life at the age of forty-nine to begin to create something that was going to be for teen girls. And honestly, Mitzi, I couldn't say yes immediately because my visions of where I was going to be as one of the next Women of Faith speakers, and then, secondary to that, did I want to go back and work with teens?

Mitzi: [Laughs]

Doreen: So that is what God was calling me to. And it was a very clear calling, and it took me three months to say yes, and God used the scripture in Esther 4:14 where it says, "You have been born for such a time as this."

Mitzi: And I'm sure you had the same thinking as myself: "We just don't have the finances" and "How am I going to do this?" or "Why am I this?" Did that occur to you?

Doreen: Of course. [Laughs] I finally did say yes because further in that verse it says if you do not respond then, I could choose someone from somewhere else.

Mitzi: Yes.

Doreen: And I thought if God's calling me, then I need

to respond or I will miss out on the blessing, but I didn't know what that blessing was going to look like until after my first Modern Day Princess celebration, of course. And in addition to that, I had an opportunity to be invited to Focus on the Family's offices shortly after saying yes to the Lord in this matter.

Mitzi: Wow.

Doreen: I had my youngest daughter come alongside with me because I had been a women's Bible study teacher for many years. But I didn't feel I had the useful perspective, and my youngest daughter had married and wasn't having to work at that time.

So she came alongside with me and created the youthful questions to provoke interaction with the teen girls throughout the curriculum. So I had the blessing of a youthful perspective from my daughter and the Biblical foundation that God had placed in my life, having been a Bible study teacher. So God brought it together in order to implement, and in fact, even have curriculum.

Mitzi: So it was all laid out, really. I mean, once you said yes, things—I mean again, not naturally in our time, natural time, but as you follow the steps it became clear and you were able to keep going to the next level or the next level—

Doreen: That's right. What was very confirming, Mitzi, was being invited to Focus on the Family's offices through a friend who used to work for Focus on the Family and who was determined that she was going to have Focus on the Family have visibility of me and the ministry. And so, she opened up those doors, and

I get a call from Focus on the Family and was invited to a summit on those who had created rite-of-passage programs for both boys and girls. And I arrived at this conference, and Mitzi, I was the only woman present at that meeting, and they were obviously focused on the family leadership, from Promise Keepers leadership and even John Trent, who wrote *The Blessing*, was present. And then other individuals such as myself who were unknown at that time. But it was amazing, Mitzi, to see that God was calling for there to be a message to the American Christian community that we needed a rite-of-passage. God had laid it on the hearts of men several years before me, but this was the first time we were actually at a summit to discuss this, and I was the only one that didn't know that I was the only one as a woman attending.

Mitzi: [Laughs] You know, it's a good thing you didn't know.

Doreen: It really was. [Laughs]

Mitzi: So, yes, Doreen—the second question is how has this endeavor changed your life plan from what you would have thought your life would look like at this age? I mean, obviously, this is much more than an endeavor. I mean, it's just this huge enterprise really, a spiritual enterprise. What had you thought, or did you have any thoughts when you were forty-nine? Did you have plans in retiring with your husband? Did you have another vision, or were you just living life, just trying to cope, and didn't really know what your future was going to look like?

Doreen: Oh, I knew the Lord had a call in my life to be

a speaker for women, and I had been developing my speaker bio before I even had been working for Women of Faith, and God called me to that role prior to the Modern Day Princess ministry. It was a confirmation that I did have a call on my life because out of all the reps that were first assigned to Women of Faith to go out and spread the news about this conference across the U.S., which we did together, I was the one chosen to speak at all of the free conference events as the emcee.

So, I thought that God had always had a call on my life just teaching Bible study, and pretty soon I'm asked to speak for a women's retreat. Then I, you know, progressed, and God opened up an incredible door, of which I've never, never applied to Women of Faith—they sought me out. And then when I was spending a lot of time with the Women of Faith speakers, Patsy Clairmont said to me at one time when I asked her, I said, "You know what, Patsy? I just finished taking Florence Littauer's CLASS and," I said, "I don't understand why I'm here." And she says, "Oh, I know exactly why you're here." I said, "Why is that?" She says, "Because we're here to mentor you." And—

Mitzi: Oh, wow.

Doreen: Was that a wow moment for me? [Laughs]

Mitzi: Oh, I would have loved to have seen your face.

Doreen: Yes, for sure, and you know what? They did take me under their wings, and you know what? Their mentorship was more on a personal level, and spending time with them both in the green room, on the floor, at their executive booths, and on stage and seeing the consistency of their vulnerability and their openness and transparency, that they were the same person before that curtain on the platform in the plane. And the transparency of their lives is what has impacted those audiences for years. And seeing that the call on their lives did not cause them to be prideful but humble, as if God was using them, I wanted that same spirit in my own life in whatever God was calling me to.

Well, you asked me, you asked me about my life plans: My life plans were that I never thought I would go back to teens, and then as life has progressed in the ministry, I had more women ask me, "Would you be willing to do this for women?" And in 2010, we created a women's curriculum that now has become just as powerful in those lives as it had to teen girls a decade before. So, we're increasing in our reach now to women and what I—my life plans, what I thought they would look like, obviously, are going back to what my first desire was, which was to be a speaker to women. And God's providing that in my own venue, just not on a Women of Faith page like I had pictured it to be. And God knows what He's doing, and I see such great fruit from it. So that's the other joy of this opportunity that He presented for me to fulfill and know that He has— He is leading me in the process.

Mitzi: Wow, yes, and so, not to put words in your mouth, Doreen, you basically never saw an ending to your working years? Or starting to really just sit out and retire like so many do. I mean, it's hard for women like you and I to imagine that, but we are the minority. And so, not to put words in your mouth but to ask you that question again. You did not see yourself as sitting on the sideline and just retiring, am I correct in that?

Doreen: That's correct.

Mitzi: Okay, that's what I thought.

Doreen: And you know, once again I take myself back to the Women of Faith, none other than Sheila Walsh, all of those women did not even start their ventures in public speaking with Women of Faith until they were between fifty and sixty years of age.

Mitzi: Oh, that just gave me goose bumps. Thank you for sharing that. [Laughs] It's awesome information for me, who just sitting here as the oldest Baby Boomer—and we love seeing in so many individuals in their later life that so many endeavors didn't start till their later years. What we want to do is encourage Boomers, especially the older ones. I just know so many who are typically purposeless and without any particular passion. Thousands upon thousands of Boomer women, especially (but men, too). Their children have grown and their husbands may or may not be retired but they're in that transition, which is huge and very perplexing, on finding their identity. They're basically asking, now what do I do with my life?

Doreen: Yeah.

Mitzi: And it's astounding to ask, isn't it, that that is happening, but it's such a lose-lose on both sides because they're losing and then all of their potential is lost.

Doreen: That's for sure. My mother, who is eighty-five, moved at least ten years ago to Santa Fe, New Mexico, to be close to Chad and I, and that was right after my

Togetherness

dad passed away. And so, she makes this major move over to Santa Fe, New Mexico, to be living close to Chad and I and my other sister. And I'm helping her unpack one day on the house, and she's pretty much at the end of all the details, and she says, "Well, now that I'm settled in my home," she says, "now, I have to find my purpose."

Mitzi: Oh, I love that.

Doreen: And I thought, wow, and interestingly enough, as she's praying about that, in the next few days a neighbor approaches her and says, "I noticed you're new in the community here and I'd just wondered if you'd be interested in participating in the foster grandparent program."

Mitzi: Oh.

Doreen: And my mother boldly says yes, and asked them if she could possibly go to our church school and be a foster grandparent there, and they said, "Yes, we're trying to get into the school, to interfaith-based organizations." And my mom—

Mitzi: Awesome.

Doreen: ...that way could work for the school two to three days a week in the library, and she found her purpose.
   Those children absolutely love my mother. She in turn couldn't wait to get to the school to organize those books and care for those children at eighty-some years of age, late seventies, early eighties, and she's still doing that.

Mitzi: Ah, and how old is she now, Doreen?

Doreen: Eighty-five.

Mitzi: Wow, and see, we're blessed because my mother, at ninety, almost ninety-one, works at the food bank. Still goes to the community center to serve the needs, and she had to pull back on other things, but she won't give that up. It's remarkable when we compare our mothers and what their lives look like, right, compared to the stereotype.

Doreen: So true.

Mitzi: Yeah, and it's going to be the same way with us Boomers, that to encourage other women at the young age, really in their late fifties, sixties, find their purpose. They have just begun in many arenas. So, that's why you're one of the inspirations for this chapter.

Doreen: One of the things that you said, "How do you feel about now at this Boomer age and what are your plans for the future as far as slowing down?"
  The only thing I can really say in that is as the responsibilities of this ministry are growing, I am learning to be able to hand off more and more of those responsibilities to others and feeling the freedom to be able to do that and not have such a fear of letting go by trusting God that he has raised up other people to come alongside of me to carry out this ministry without me.

Mitzi: This thing to let go. I mean, you have the willingness to just open your hands and say, okay.

Doreen: Yes. I said, "I love doing it," but I realized there are other responsibilities that I have if I'm going to write two other books, which Focus on the Family asked us to write for Little Princesses and one for women now.

So, the reality is, if I'm going to take on those endeavors, I've got to let go of others, and God put a very confident woman before me to take over something that I really love and would love to continue doing, but I need to lay down something in order to do the other. [Laughs]

Mitzi: Well, the last question, because I know you're a busy, busy lady, is we touched on how so many hundreds of thousands of Boomers, who are my passion and purpose in my heart, are hurting. They're sad and they're lonely and isolated and purposeless. I know that we can say to them just get out there—and it's not a platitude, we truly mean that. But is there—are there more concrete things that you could encourage and advise women to do? And I know Boomer men, too, face these life crossroads, and "What would I do now?" But we're aiming at women like you are. So—

Doreen: I think God is always looking for opportunities for us to be able to serve Him and some other—it can be the most simple thing of offering to pray for somebody to providing a ride or a meal, and God has a purpose for our lives. And I think sometimes we're blind to it because we're so self-focused, like hurting, "I'm lonely," "We don't have any money," "We don't…" You know. And yet, God has opportunities for us every day to bless others, and when we take the focus off of ourselves and look for opportunities to volunteer and bless others, we're going to begin to develop a legacy whether with—maybe their family legacy or spiritual legacy. We have the opportunity to do that if we'll just look to see how we can meet the needs of others. And I know—here's a good example. There are homeless people that beg every day at a corner where I have to turn on to get onto the freeway, and I was discouraged when my husband says, "You know, I don't want you giving them money every day. They're not using it for good things," and you know. Well, we need to do something, you know. [Laughs] And so, I talked to my daughter, and I said, "You know what? What do you think about us getting a little quart-size Ziploc bag. I'll buy the water or I'll buy the goodies." And then our six-year-old granddaughter, who loves to write, she's just learning to write, on the back of a simple million-dollar play money note—the back of it is blank—she, in her little handwriting, would write, "We're praying for you." And on the front side is a track of how we need Christ compared to a million dollars, of course. So, that little track, her little handwriting, a small bottle of water and some crackers or cookies or something, it's helped. So great knowing that we were meeting a need.

Mitzi: Yes and it—again, it's out of you and it's not a big deal as far as what it costs you.

Doreen: That's right.

Mitzi: That's a beautiful example, Doreen. You said it very eloquently. It's so much nicer than what I wrote in part of this chapter. What I said, what I wrote was, "Get over yourself." [Laughs]

Doreen: [Laughs] Well, that's about right, Mitzi. That's exactly what it is. [Laughs]

Mitzi: Oh, I can see that how, just thoughtful and sweet

you are versus Mitzi. [Laughs]

Doreen: Well, some people need it said that way, Mitzi. That's the truth of why God has you say it that way. [Laughs]

Mitzi: Togetherness…giving back…leaving a legacy…being a positive influence…you are most definitely all of these, Doreen, and many, many Boomers will be enlightened and encouraged by all you shared and all you are doing. Thank you!

Chapter 6
Spirituality

Connecting the Dots: How Boomer Smarts Enables Boomers to Live in Boomer Power

Two Types of Boomer Power

Now is the time for you Boomers to decide if I am going to be your best friend or your worst enemy with the information in this book. And, of course, you have probably figured out by now that I am not going away to Never Never Land not to be seen or heard from again. Oh no!

Whoever you decide I am, friend or foe, I cannot complete this manuscript without fully explaining what Boomer Power actually is.

So now, let's define and differentiate what I mean by living with and in Boomer Power.

This is a twofold entity. One most definitely means that living with Boomer Smarts will propel us light years ahead of those Boomers who continue to remain the same year after year, not preparing for their futures.

I accept the fact that millions of Boomers may not believe in God or a higher power, but nevertheless, they can have the remarkable opportunity to live their Boomer years ahead with Boomer Power from living with the Boomer Smart principles to age better and age smarter.

The second meaning of Boomer Power, for me personally, is the most essential power that comes from our faith. For example:

I have been asked so many times since buying Cypress, which was in such deplorable condition, "Why this house?" Well, I still struggle with how to explain the unexplainable to most people. To say that I just knew this was our house makes no sense in our rational, logical way of processing life-changing decisions. But this is the only response I have to all those inquiring minds. I just knew this was our house. How we were going to accomplish this huge undertaking is another question—I had absolutely no idea. I only knew that I knew we were to do this crazy, irrational, life-changing restoration, believe it or not, because God said so. This is the power I am referring to as the second type of Boomer Power that comes from our faith.

I must and just have to digress here, so forgive me, dear Boomers. To those that do understand what I mean by this last paragraph on my faith, let me perhaps further blow your mind. We never saw the inside of this house before we made an offer to buy. But before Bob and I walked through it the very first time—in the mess, and garbage, and filth—I told him exactly where all the rooms would be and what they would look like. Now how could I possibly know this space-planning layout before seeing the inside? Again, believe it or not, but I know the Lord told me exactly what was to happen—and ask Bob, this is exactly what indeed did happen for the interior rooms of Cypress. This is faith from the power...not by might nor by power but by His Spirit.

Connect the Dots

The chapter concepts in my writing for this book on

Spirituality

Space, Mindset, Attitudes, Routines, Togetherness, and Spirituality represent the tip of the iceberg, of course, on what is yet to be discovered on the aging Boomer. Obvious, also, is the fact that I could only partially write about health, home, and attitudes as, of course, there are literally volumes of material on each one of these major topics.

But the main thing is the main thing, and that is how essential it is that we Boomers do get, understand, and put into practice these Boomer Smart principles in our daily Boomer lives. The entire Boomer Smart message to achieve the ultimate Boomer Power can be summed up in two words: GET PREPARED!

What good is it to be really working hard on healthy lifestyles only to slip and fall in the bathroom, leading to major and long-lasting chronic issues, such as a back or head injury, for example. Or what good is it to say yes, embracing the research that expounds that our attitudes and mindsets do affect our aging, but we still continue an unhealthy lifestyle? No, we must incorporate all three areas to live wisely in our best rest years and CONNECT THE DOTS!

Boomer Smarts concepts are based on three basic areas to achieve the Boomer Power living we all want and deserve.

our ATTITUDES   our LIFESTYLES   our HOMES

All of the Boomer Smarts principles are wrapped up in these big three. Therefore, get prepared in your attitude, your lifestyle, and your home for what is the inevitable fact of life: AGING.

But no worries, though, really, since Boomers who are aging with a Boomer Smart ATTITUDE readily handle and accept this aging as an inevitable fact of life. That is why we are the Smart Boomers!

Think of a three-legged stool, with each leg representing either our attitudes, our lifestyles, or our homes. Take away one of the legs and what happens? No stability; it's wobbly and weak. All three legs in place provide stability, security, and strength.

Remember, my dear fellow Boomers, all of life is a choice. Yes, ALL OF LIFE IS A CHOICE in what we think about things, how we talk about things, and how we do things in our daily lives.

So pat yourself on the back if you are now considering how you will choose to spend your future best rest years. Even this one small step of thinking about your future puts you way above most Boomers.

I predict that if you are now thinking and considering your daily choices, your life is going to change for the better. You'll see.

Millions of Boomers Were Hurt by
Their Religious Upbringing

As we have been expounding on how much America has and is changing since we Boomers have been born, especially the older Boomers, our culture has seen the biggest changes, without a doubt.

It is hard for my grandchildren to even believe we had to actually get out of our chair to change the TV channel! And speaking of TV, I vividly remember Ozzie and Harriet and other major TV stars in twin beds on the rare shots we even saw them in their bedrooms.

And on going to church, well, it was the odd or an unusual family that didn't attend church or at least take their kids and drop them off at Sunday school. Some of my most fun times in junior high were going to whatever church youth group was having a dance or hay ride

Spirituality

or roller-skating party. I was there and so were all my friends, no matter what church they went to, if even they went at all.

Boomer Power stems from Boomer Smarts enlightened by a spiritual relationship, not of laws or religion.

However, now in America, the Pew Research polls tell us that it is the minority of Americans who are attending church. Our culture has all but said "we do not need religion anymore." And surprise surprise, I do not think we need religion, either, if it is a dogma of rules and guilt-producing religious practices. But without a doubt, I believe we need to believe and have a sustaining faith that comes from a relationship with the Lord...not living under the law of rules and guilt-producing dogma. "The traditions of man make the word of God null and void of original intent."

Those Boomers formerly hurt by their religious past are now empowered and are seeking and finding their true Boomer Power in Him.

And yet millions of Americans are finding this relationship in their churches or in small groups or just in themselves. But they are indeed finding it again, especially as the world gets crazier and crazier and, it seems, more unpredictable almost daily. The difference to me in a sustaining faith is again quite simple. It gives my life purpose. My personal belief is that if we truly are believers, our lives show it in intentional living and giving to others. It is not about the "bless my four and no more."

Boomer Power comes from the Boomer Smarts that our Creator is the true Power.

And this is the power that I depend on over and over again in my day-by-day busy life. But whenever I get discouraged, overwhelmed, down, or frustrated, I've learned I'm looking at the now...the situation...the circumstance. And if or when my thinking agrees with what I see, I lose hope that things will ever change or get better. This is exactly when I need to look in God's Word, not at what is in front of me in any given situation or every crisis or just plain everyday living.

"Our house isn't selling. What do we do now?" "The basement foundation is so cracked at Cypress and it is falling in. Can it truly be repaired? And how much will this cost?" "What? The Realtor is showing between four and six today." "The basement stairs will need to take more of the dining area." "So what will we do to place our beautiful antique furniture" "What? The subs didn't show up again? How are we ever going to finish this house?"

The Hardest Test

To persevere by hanging on when there appears to be no reason to hope—this is the hardest part of our faith, which was absolutely the case in trying to finish Cypress. Add to this hopelessness people's opinions, criticisms, doubts, and gossip, and we can slime ourselves with yesterday's mold and grime all over again.

"Boy, Cypress sure is taking a long time."

"Did you see the mess Bob and Mitzi bought?"

"I heard Mitzi's business is down the tubes. What is she doing?"

"Why would they buy this horribly run-down house at their age?"

This is why doubt, fear, and insecurities are the true tests of the depth of our faith. Yes, I have lost many of these tests over the past years, but now I have seen more victories by my faith than I could possibly convey in this book. And the good news is that even with the tests that I may fail in the future, my hope in His unconditional love allows me and encourages me to get up and try again.

Spirituality

Authentic Boomer Power from authentic faith has compassion and love for fellow Boomers, not judgment and criticism. One of the saddest changes I see in America today is our loss of tolerance for those that believe or think differently than we do. If you knew how many friends I have that are atheists, gay, liberal, ultra-conservative, or agnostic, you would be very surprised. And these friends of mine, in turn, respect what I believe, which in many areas is totally opposite of what they believe or do not believe. This is what's so special about my friends. We allow each other to have our own beliefs without judging or criticizing.

Unfortunately, tolerance in America today really means you have to agree with me or you are a bigot. My goodness. How sad for America that we have come to this point. And this is exactly why, again, I personally believe so many Boomers left the church and will never darken another church door again. I hope and pray that, as Boomers, they will know us by our love, even with those with whom we disagree.

Without Hope, Faith is Impossible

Everyone believes in something. Think about it—self, others, career, etc. What are you putting your hope in? Your investments, your inheritance, your 401K, your company's security, your health, your spouse's income?

Yes, we all have to believe in something or someone, as these Boomers in the following scenarios did. Man oh man, what happened is another tragedy all too common, as Boomers are experiencing them by the zillions it seems.

One couple in their mid-sixties had very successful careers that gave them a wonderful retirement. Until one day it all came crumbling down. They had invested their retirement with a financial planner that embezzled their nest egg.

A friend in her sixties found out her very well-known and very successful husband of over forty-five years has had an affair and now wants a divorce. It is a very ugly divorce, and it's astonishing that income and investments can be hidden so deep that truly the only winners are the divorce attorneys as they battle for disclosures that seem to never happen.

Another dear, dear friend, late sixties, is married to a wonderful man who has had much success in his own business and had a stellar reputation with everyone. So it came as a great shock when my friend found out their money had all but disappeared. Her husband had developed Alzheimer's, evidently, while in his fifties but was undiagnosed until years and years later. His behavior at home, for the most part, was his normal behavior. Eventually, it became clear that something was terribly wrong with this wonderful and so-loved man. Money gone, future unknown.

And as we all know and see, Baby Boomers with the best of planning are still not secure, as life does happen in ways no one expects. This explains why droves of Boomers are reevaluating their beliefs based on lives that have not worked out as they planned, in a world seemingly out of control, with economic instabilities abounding, families torn apart or at odds, and on and on.

But this book is on getting Boomer Smarts to empower us with Boomer Power in our future best rest years, so why all this doom and gloom? Well, how can we not be realists when the lives I've described could happen to any one of us?

I maintain unequivocally, though, that with practiced and mastered Boomer Smarts, if and when life hits us broadside, we will without a doubt be so much better

Spirituality

off and prepared than those scrambling around in their oh-my-goodness state of compromised coping with their latest issue or crisis.

No, it is all the more imperative to be prepared for what may happen…or may not. But if it should happen, those with an abiding faith will weather their storms with their sustaining faith that keeps them going and keeps them strong. I have witnessed this dozens and dozens and dozens of times.

This chapter, however, is on my own spirituality, and in no way do I judge anyone else's faith or views or positions on this very hot topic. Am I just being politically correct here?

No, I am attempting to be nonjudgmental because as I judge, I will be judged.

What I dearly love about our God is that He gives us free choice. Never ever are we dominated or forced into believing in the One True One. Every single person alive decides or chooses what to believe or not believe. It is simply that simple.

The building years for our restored 1930s home we call Cypress were years and years of doubt, fear, and anxiety. Years full of a lot of tension and uncertainty of how we would ever get back on our feet financially.

Remember, we were all set to finally get set for "the now is our time" for Mitzi and Bob's financial future to start building up…finally!! Then, shocked, I asked Bob, "What, your job was eliminated?"

Well, it only takes a few years of nonworking to drain one's financial security, especially when those were to be the buildup years and not the drain years. And might I add that we were in our mid-fifties! It doesn't take a math genius to figure out this one; we didn't have many years left to prepare for a secure future.

As we watched our friends taking world cruises, driving beautiful cars, and basically leading the life most Boomers had hoped for and truthfully expected, Bob and I were basically sucking air trying to survive in our later Boomer years.

But my faith said, "Hang in there, Mitzi, keep on keeping on and have hope that all is well and all will be well."

I know, I know; this is so easy to say but so hard to actually do in everyday struggles. But I told myself, "You can do it afraid, Mitzi, but just do something!"

Where We Are Now

So now what is the status of Bob and Mitzi? Well, we are living an exciting and satisfying life. We are both enjoying excellent health...not perfect but definitely excellent. Our three adult children are married, each with three beautiful children, living successful lives. We are absolutely and totally beyond loving and living in our home, Cypress. I am still working my interior design business and Bob is still working in the oil refinery business. Our lives are very busy with travel, careers, and just living life. We have been married for forty-five years, and I always say, that's amazing grace! But this all did not come without years of paying a huge price in time, effort, money, and, of course, prayer. No, we did not just land here, and no, of course our life is not perfect...but it is good... very good.

One last "time," *times are changing in America!* An untold number of Baby Boomers want or have had to reinvent themselves as their situations change or they change in wanting to do more or do something totally different with their lives.

A major part of having Boomer Smarts is recognizing the changes going on in our individual careers, and the field of interior design has been no exception to this major change. I have had to reinvent the way I do my design business many, many times over the past ten years due to HGTV, the Internet, showroom policy changes, consumers' new and often unrealistic attitudes on wanting the absolute bottom price with the absolute best design service—and oh, by the way, they want it yesterday!

This never used to be the way it was, as we designers were much more appreciated rather than being seen as a means to someone's end. I love my clients who appreciate how hard I work for them with all the experience and knowledge that I can possibly put forth in their projects. My clients see and know that I strive to make each home, to the best of my designer's ability, a home that embraces their lifestyles in function, comfort, and beauty. However, there is no perfect project, and I am certainly not a perfect interior designer!

So in my Boomer Smarts, observing all these major changes in my profession, for years I have known being a full-time professional interior designer was not going to be my life. I have known that I know there is another calling, passion, dream to fulfill in this next stage of Boomer life.

But to get there is a, "What, are you kidding me, how are you possibly going to do that?"

You guessed right if you said by faith. My faith over these many years has sustained me in the hope that where a serious passion and life path is planted, in order to complete one's life purpose, that dream must come to fruition. This is where the majority fail to realize their passions/dreams/plans/next career by looking at their own strengths, their own resources, their own age, their own abilities.

Along with continuing my interior design business in some form, my mission, so to speak, is to speak to Baby Boomers on preparing themselves for what is next in their health and their homes, as we have covered in these last chapters.

Nice idea, Mitzi, but how in tarnation do you expect to do this? Beats me. I only knew that I knew I was to do this, and my faith told me to do what I had to do one step at a time.

Now this has been my journey for *many* years of long, lonely, and hard work simply because I believed this is what I can absolutely accomplish through His strength, His power, not mine. But the battle was fierce in my thoughts of doubt, fear, anxiety, and insecurity.

It is so easy to say, "I am too old, I don't have the experience, I don't have the skills or seriously doubt spending money at this stage of life on a total unknown outcome." Herein lies the biggest battle there is to moving into our future destiny as a Baby Boomer.

I had to believe that I am a writer, that I am a speaker, that I will make a difference in Baby Boomers' lives. I had to believe that I will learn technical skills to accomplish these goals, and on and on. But what was I basing all my belief on? The Lord and His strength and His power, not mine. I had literally no one to help me do this crazy, unrealistic, unheard of dream, but I had to stand on my faith that He would bring those people to me, and indeed He has.

Overcoming our mental battles by faith in our beliefs, to me, is the only answer. Every day, for years and years and years, I have started my day in a devotional sharing with the Lord. This is the ONLY reason I am where I am. I did not have the skills, experience, finances, and certainly I did not have youth on my side, but I believed preparing Baby Boomers with Boomer Smarts to live their best life is my purpose.

And now it is paying off.

Here is my secret to where I am and where I am going.

Spirituality

Boomer Power

Where does this Boomer Power come from? Well, we obviously know by now that this Boomer Power comes by getting the Boomer Smarts that equip and enlighten us to move always forward in preparing for our futures. My Boomer Power, however, is sustained by a Boomer Power in Him.

But knowledge is power, and getting more knowledge is always empowering in gaining the wisdom so necessary for achieving understanding. Then the "aha!" moments come to connect the dots on "oh, this is why I need to do this or this is why I need to have that."

I realize, of course, that many do not share the same faith as me, and for all those Baby Boomers the message is still the same—get knowledge, get wisdom, get understanding to get Boomer Smarts to live the very best that life can possibly bring.

A profound scripture to me is in Hosea, which says, "My people perish for lack of knowledge." Therein lies my whole purpose for my beloved and fellow Boomers. To share the knowledge that I have been given to motivate, educate, and inspire Boomers in preparing their health and homes to become empowered with life-sustaining BOOMER POWER.

No one can do this for us, but once obtained, no one can take it away from us, either.

Watch and see. You will without a doubt spot in a nanosecond those Boomers who have indeed obtained this Boomer Smart lifestyle driven by Boomer Power.

A Baby Boomer living in and with Boomer Power will be a beacon of light for their families, friends, colleagues, communities, and who knows...maybe even the world! You'll see.

Boomer Smart Stories

Leslie Wood
Hadley Court
www.HadleyCourt.com

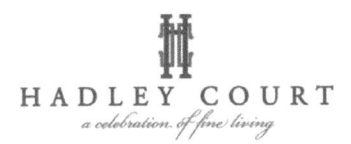

HADLEY COURT
a celebration of fine living

Mitzi: The purpose of the book is to inspire, educate, and motivate Baby Boomers, and our target market is those in their mid forties and into their sixties. The Baby Boomers were born between 1946 and 1964. So, as of 2013, the youngest are fifty, the oldest are sixty-seven. And they are the biggest, wealthiest, and often the most educated, powerful group in America right now.

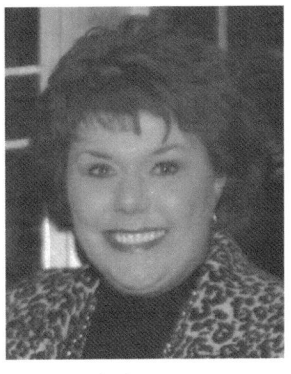

But what I'm seeing, and I'm sure you observed and witnessed it also, is that things are changing so quickly and drastically in America that one, either the Baby Boomers are totally not aware living in this naivety bubble, or two, they do know what is happening but they do not have a clue how to move forward or how to prepare.

So, in the book, the chapters form the acronym S.M.A.R.T.S. as chapter topics. S is Spaces. M is for Mindsets. A is for Attitudes. R is for Routines or lifestyle. T is Togetherness, which is living a legacy, being out of ourselves, giving back. And S is for Spiritual. And that's where you come in.

Just from reading your blog, I know that your faith is a part of your life. So, the first question I have for you,

Spirituality

Leslie, is how has your faith influenced your present Boomer life stage?

Leslie: I think my faith has allowed me to focus on what I think are the most important things in my life. Number one, God. Number two, family. And then beyond that is helping your community and then your occupation. So, it has helped me order my life in ways I think are God-centered.

Mitzi: Okay, well said, Leslie. I love that your faith helped you focus your life. And as far as your Boomer life stage right now, having your faith be part of who you are, you're very comfortable with that, it appears.

Leslie: Yes, I am. As far as my faith, I am very comfortable with my faith. I'm not—I guess it's kind of a quiet faith. I don't feel the need to scream it from the house tops, you know.
 I think one of the biggest things of believing in God is to let that shine through you, by the way you live. And you don't necessarily have to scream it to people. You just need to live it and it shines through.

Mitzi: Yes, and you know, I struggled with the book, being a Christian, and it's the most important thing in my life. I wanted the spiritual aspect to be part of the book because it's part of becoming and living in wholeness and balance.

Leslie: Right, uh huh.

Mitzi: And I really have struggled with how much to be specific or how, you know, how—where is the line, because there are so many people we love and care about that we know if they pick up and see scriptures or something, then they put it down just as quickly.

Leslie: Right.

Mitzi: And so, I have decided, through a lot of prayer, now that I'm putting it out there in a, not like you said, a scream, but in a quiet way—

Leslie: Uh huh.

Mitzi: ...but it will be known and—but I've also done a lot of explanation that there are different faiths and there are different ways, but this is my own personal point of view and so forth. So, you know, I agree with you, but yet, I don't hide it. It would be wrong for me. I would be in disobedience if I did this book, and I'm talking about the six steps to living a Boomer life that's filled with Boomer Power, and not reveal what my biggest power is, you know, which is—

Leslie: Right.

Mitzi: ...my faith. So—

Leslie: Right. I agree. And—

Mitzi: Okay. So—

Leslie: ...I think if—I think, you know, everybody is at a different stage and if—I think if you go about it kind of quietly and just leave...leave the message there that if and when they're ready to hear it, they will, you know.

Mitzi: That's a good point. And that it's about acceptance, which is part of the chapter. This chapter on spirituality is about being non-judgmental, non-critical toward others, and that really is the faith walk. However, in America today, that if we are not in agreement, we are considered intolerant. And that's not the way our faith works. We just have a different belief system.

Leslie: Right.

Mitzi: Let's talk about that a little bit, that our faith is for acceptance of everyone and we hope that respect is unconditional, meaning simply respecting the person from whatever point of view they come from.

Since there are so many that are lost, so to speak, with so much that has happened in America, this is the second question to you. Millions of Boomers losing jobs and all kinds of things happening to this demographic that no other generation before has experienced. Our parents' lives were pretty predictable in many ways. But for the Baby Boomers, we're the pioneer adding in to this. We're talking about those that are struggling and how many people are really at crossroads and do not know how to reposition themselves. What advice can you give to help? Their lives are goings off track, whether it's health or finance or in a divorce or whatever it might be that are struggling. Do you have any words of wisdom?

Leslie: Well, you know, I think we've all faced hardship, and actually I have, which I'm not really public about, but I, you know, I have chosen to rise above that, and every day is a new day. And I think, of course, faith has a lot to do with that. But especially in America, anything is possible, and it's just all about what to tell yourself every day if it's going to be a good day or a bad day. And you just have to carry on, I think. And the bottom line, no matter what your resources are, I think if you have the love of your family and believe in God, then I think things are manageable. I think you can get through the tough times.

Mitzi: I think you hit on the key point. It is the love of family that certainly brings many through the tough times, but it's shocking to hear the statistics on singles today. I was talking to Cynthia Bogart of the Daily Basics; she was one of the regional editors for *Better Homes & Gardens*. She is married and has a family, but she said the statistic she just heard was seventy percent of America is single. And that shocked me. I heard, the last I was aware of, it was fifty percent. So for those without a lot of family, I'm sure our advice to them is going to be we have to prepare ahead of time, right, with a social family with those we built up in a support system before the bottom falls out or before we retire or whatever.

Leslie: Right. Yes.

Mitzi: So, how does your faith impact your future plans? As you have a design business, you have your blog and other writing and whatnot, how do you see the interaction of your blog and your faith? I mean—and does your faith influence your business?

Leslie: Oh, absolutely. You know, I am—I have a business degree, actually, and a master's in business and a background in business. And I was basically groomed to take over my family's oil business and things didn't work out with my dad and I very well. And so, I chose to stay home with my children. I had that opportunity, and I chose that, and because I wanted—no matter what—whatever my children turned out to be, I wanted to know that I had done the best job I possibly could. And so, it's about reevaluating and identifying on and off throughout the years my interest and talent in interior design but it was just here and there but not steadily. And about two years ago, I just had this epiphany that I had, sort of, I've always been very creative that I sort of get interior design—my father didn't view that as worthy.

And I sort of pushed it under the rug. But then, I had an epiphany that by doing so, I was snubbing God. That was the greatest gift he had given me, my talent and creativity, and I wasn't using it, and I was basically turning my back on him. So that's when I decided to start my—start designing, you know, more. My kids are older now. They're almost eighteen and fifteen, and so I started working, and my business has just been thriving, and it's more of a full-time business right now. It's kind of the same thing with the blog, I had no—I mean, the blog does not bring me design business.

Mitzi: No, I understand it.

Leslie: But it was like I just felt the drive that I had to… to start this blog for whatever reason.

Mitzi: I can relate to that one!

Leslie: And so, I have and I just—I feel like it's God-led. I'm really not sure what the purpose is or why, but I mean that's really the reason for the blog, and I think, like me winning that award, that was simply God. I mean there's tons of great design blogs out there, you know? So, whatever He has in store for me with this,

I'm not sure, but—

Mitzi: I love it.

Leslie: So, He's got a big, big impact.

Mitzi: And you've listened. I mean, it's easy to have that push, that nudge you feel led someday to do, but those of us, and I'm saying this humbly, it aint easy, is it? Because it's very scary to actually do it. But if I'll get out there and be among those who stepped out and do the whatever is next, well, we are also blessed that we didn't hold back

Leslie: Right. Well, it's a very uncomfortable—I think maybe sometimes when you're not using God's gift, there's a real unsettling feeling.

Mitzi: Yes.

Leslie: You're not necessarily whole or complete—maybe it wasn't necessarily obvious always, and you didn't know why, but I feel really comfortable where I am right now, and I think it has a lot to do that I'm using His gift.

Mitzi: Uh huh, absolutely. They say when we're in our gift thing, life just flows. And that's what I'm hearing you say. And I just have to share this with you, that you and I would have never met had we not been bloggers. I was sitting down behind you when you won the award, and I went, "Wow, that's her!" I'm thinking, because I was a newbie and still am, but it was just— it made it real to me, that people can do this and it's not about being twenty-eight and not that you're one

Spirituality

of the older Boomers, but it is. It's just about stepping out and doing what we think we're supposed to be doing. And we don't have to have the answers, do we? We don't have to know the purpose, so to speak, which is we're just doing it. So—

Leslie: Uh huh, right. Well, it's kind of like Noah and his Ark, you know, he just did it having no clue what would be next, but he knew he just had to do it.

Mitzi: Perfect ending, Leslie. Thank you for your sharing your wisdom so beautifully.

Karen Porter
Bold Vision Books
www.BoldVisionBooks.com

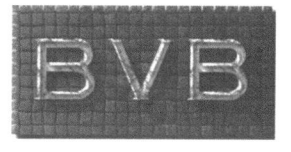

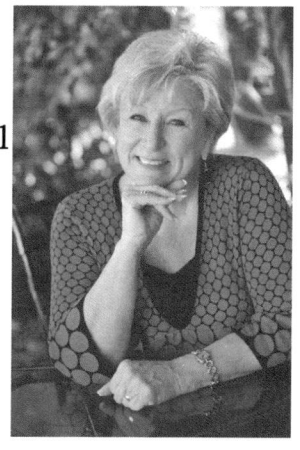

Mitzi: Okay. Well, the reason I have asked you to do one of the interviews for the book was your story on how your life was—versus how your actual life currently is—that you so powerfully shared at the CLASS Houston Speakers Conference. And there are just hundreds of thousands of Baby Boomers out there that had similar situations, as you're aware of them, of course. And so the purpose of the spiritual chapter of the book is, how do we use our faith to redirect us? There is no simple answer, I understand, but I hope we can share with other Boomers out there who have had to face life situations that took them off their life plan for their futures.

Karen: Exactly.

Mitzi: Okay. So, the first question for you, Karen, is what was your significant life event and what was your response to this event that changed your Boomer path of what you had anticipated your life to be?

Karen: Okay, I was in the corporate world for thirty-three years. I worked for a major food company, and in that thirty-three years, I worked my way up through the ranks from just working in a marketing department to eventually becoming vice president in charge of International Marketing. And in that job, I was involved in branding and developing markets all over the world, and that was quite challenging because some markets are very modern markets, like we have here in the United States, and other markets are very primitive.

And there are all kinds of cultural questions and that kind of thing that go with that. And so I was able—at some point, you know, at some places where we sold the product, we might sell a shipload to go into a place where food products were, people were desperate for food, and other places, we sold in small packages just like you'd see at your local grocery store.

So, it's a broad range of things, and I had worked my way to the top, and I had sort of made it, I thought, and I was in—for me personally, it was very important to be in on the development of the company, the future of the company, to be in on the decision-making, to, you know, to develop what the company would become. And so, I had reached that point and I was in the inside track, in the know. And we had gone through a number of different challenges in our industry and in our business over the course of those years. But at one point we were purchased by a foreign company, and it was very exciting for us because they had had such success with other companies, and we thought it was a great future for us.

And so, there I sat at my desk, thinking that the future looked great and bright, and I was very excited. And anyway, I got called in to the president's office one morning not knowing a thing, knowing that—thinking that they just wanted their morning reports and that sort of thing. And when I went there, the president of the company said, "I'm sorry to tell you this, but your job has been eliminated."

Mitzi: Wow.

Karen: And so, after thirty-three years, and building myself up to that place, I lost—I mean the job was gone. It wasn't—it had nothing really to do with what I'd done. It's just that that's what they did. They managed their company from Europe and they did not want you as management in there.

Mitzi: Wow.

Karen: Eventually, everyone lost their job there, but I was the first. And it—I'll tell you, for me, it was not so much losing the job, because I mean I could work anywhere, but it was a great loss of identity because I didn't—I had worked so hard to get to where I was. I almost didn't know who I was other than the corporate Karen, you know?

So it was very hard, and it did completely change our lives.

Mitzi: And so, how then did you reset your life—going off the track, so to speak, to where you are at now? And if I remember correctly, you just had built your dream home, is that—was that—

Karen: That is right. We had just built it a couple of years before; we had planned and saved and dreamed and bought a large piece of property at some acreage and we had built this home that had been twenty years in the making and the dreaming of it. And we had everything in that home that you could ever imagine wanting. It was the perfect place and we were there about five years; well, about four years, I think, before this happened to me at my job.

So, when this happened then, there I was without a job, and so the first thing we had to do was sell that house.

Mitzi: Wow.

Karen: And having only been there a few years, you can imagine that we were turned upside down by it all. It was also when the first of the downturn for housing went on, the bottom fell out the first time. And so we had no buyers. We had no buyers for a while, but then we eventually, over the course of time, we got three bids on it, and all three of them fell through for various reasons—either the people got cold feet because of the market or whatever. So we finally sold it and had to leave, to come out of that house, and there was a lot of grieving that went on with that.

Mitzi: So much—

Karen: I can't—well, you know, I remember that I was

Spirituality

grieving a great deal about the job, of the identity, and then now the house. And so, we determined to move away from that area to another part; we lived in the Houston, Texas, area. And so, we were way, way north of Houston in a fairly exclusive area, and we decide to move south of Houston to be close to one of our children. And so, the only thing to do at that point was to rent a house, which after you lived in your dream home, renting a house is the most humbling and horrible experience of all.

And I finally found a house and moved in and I just went about grieving. My husband was still working, and I just thought about grieving about that, and I had so much stuff from that big house to move in to this small house, and it was just everywhere. So that contributed to my misery, if you want to know the truth; but anyway, a remarkable thing began to happen to me. The day that I had lost my job, I discovered a verse in Psalms; after crying and wailing all day, thinking I was going to die because of this terrible thing, I came across this verse in a Psalm that says, "You will not die." And so that was like a thing that I did really cling to the whole time. And I went to this new house and I began to, you know, just sit around and grieve. I'd never in my whole life stayed at home. So, that was a horrible experience for me. And I felt really useless. And then a remarkable thing happened, which I can only credit to God Himself.

I got a phone call one day from an agency of the State of Texas asking if I was available to do some editing for them. They do a lot of research, and they needed someone to edit the report. And they would send them to me digitally and I could do the editing. And the only thing was that this person who was in charge of that, some years before, she just mentioned that, "I have a friend that might be able to do that for me." And it was a hand of God.

And so, anyway, to make the long story short, I sat in my pajamas and did that work and was paid to do that work, which was very cathartic and healing for me to be able to do work and be paid, but yet still be able to sort of recoup and grieve over everything.

And then as I did that job—and I stayed with that, doing that for a couple of years—I began to take on clients who needed help with writing and speaking because I was doing both at the time. And so, eventually, I started a company to do writing and speaking, coaching for people, which just developed into all kinds of wonderful opportunities. Then two years ago, that company evolved into a publishing company, which my husband and I started. So, resetting is a really good way to put it in your question because we basically did, you know, reset our lives, and since then—just to talk about the house, we moved from that rental house to a house that was provided for us in a kind of a miraculous way, but again smaller, then to a smaller house, and now we're even in a smaller house. But we have let go of everything. We gave away thousands of books. We gave away furniture. We gave away stuff, and it is the most freeing, wonderful thing to be—

Mitzi: Beautiful.

Karen: ...sort of in control of all of our stuff and it's not controlling us anymore. So, that's been an extra bonus thing. But now we're busy as ever, and we're running our own business and no one can come in and say our job has been eliminated.

Mitzi: Wow. You are...you are totally the Boomer's suc-

Spirituality

cess story as far as landing on your feet and finding something that you dearly—not only do you love, but you have a passion to reach out for other people and—

Karen: Yeah, I love that, and I love that place that I'm in, but I really don't want to minimize what I went through to get here because it was a terrible grieving process. But I think the key to it all is to—is first of all an abiding faith that you know that the worst thing that happened to you is no surprise to God, and the second thing is that you—you have an opportunity to look up and to say there is light. There is something out there, and then whatever gets put in your path, you take advantage of it. And so—I mean you—I could have wallowed in there forever and just become a bitter woman, you know. And I could have sued, I could have done a lot of things, but I chose to just make my life, you know, to start over. And so, I love that, and that's what people have to do.

You have to build on something and just let it go and then figure out what you're going to do for the future because I don't want to—I didn't want to sue because I don't want to wallow in it. And I didn't want to, you know, whine about it because that's wallowing in it. I wanted to move on. And I'm actually aware that positive attitude came from my faith.

Mitzi: Oh, yes. Okay. Karen, can I ask you how old you were when the bottom fell out of your life plan?

Karen: I was fifty-nine.

Mitzi: Wow. Okay.

Karen: So, yeah. So, you know that is—It's terrible. It's

terrible. I was fifty-nine, and what was I going to do? It's a terrible thing to do to anybody.

Mitzi: It is, and I say this generically because it's what we hear and see, that most people in their fifties and early sixties, when things like this happen, many really crash and burn, retreat inward, because they think there is no other path. They believe there is no other course for them to reset and rework their life. And that's the whole purpose of this interview and this book, to encourage others. And so, the last question for you is this: Does your faith impact your future plans in business and other endeavors?

Karen: Yeah, but in a way that I didn't expect.

Mitzi: Oh?

Karen: That's a good question because I expected—I mean, with my faith being part of my background and being part of how I've lived my life, you would think that's what I would say. Oh, there's—you know, I would just have faith in God. But the difference is—I don't know exactly how to say it. The difference is that, well, during those years I worked so hard to get where I got in the business world. And I had faith in God, but I also had great faith in me because I was capable in doing this on and on like that. And now, I have now, I have less faith in me and more in Him, if that makes sense. I mean, I'm just willing to let Him bring the next thing that comes along. And it's really worked beautifully in our lives, as we started this publishing company because we started out with one potential client, and that's developed into another, and you know, I sit here today, In front of me is a potential fairly big piece of business that could change everything, but we did not pursue it. It just—it came because I think I'm more or less—well, I know I am more dependent on Him than I ever was before. And I don't know if that makes sense, but I think—

Mitzi: It does, all of it.

Karen: I think anything that would have happened before, I would have probably proudly taken some credit for it. But—

Mitzi: Uh huh, okay. Well, what you said about why I said that key is when you're starting on this train of thought, you said that you have to have confidence in yourself, and as you ended this train of thought, you gave credit and glory to God. But when I said key is because I think us Boomers have to have that initial faith in ourselves, you know, and obviously coming from His power in us, but we can't move forward if we don't have faith that we are worthy—

Karen: That's very true.

Mitzi: ...and we can move on, and yes, we may step in our hole, but we know who's going to bring us up. But it has to start that inner, what-you-knew-you-had ability, and you knew that you did have thirty-three years of corporate life and that you did indeed have skill. And I think that's key, Karen, and I appreciate that thought. Well, all of this is powerful, and I'm just more than grateful that you were so authentic and shared your story.

Epilogue
What's Next?

I want to thank you, my dear Boomer friend, for reading along and joining me on this journey. The contents of this book have been my passion for a number of years and I'm so very pleased to have shared them with you and so many others.

But this idea of Boomers leading the charge to change aging in America is not just an idea. Oh no, it is really happening and we are going to be the ones to lead the charge!

How do Boomers get started and become part of this Boomer movement?

Well, if you really want to get to your next level, I will help you live the best rest of your life. We want to get together on this and I want to help you get there.

Whether it's a blog post, an interview, a webinar, or a link to a resource, my goal will be to equip you with everything you need to live your best for the rest of your life!

Join me on my site www.MitziBeach.com, where I publish blog posts and social media updates daily. I want to hear from you how you are doing and what questions you have! This is not a one-way conversation. I want to dialog with you who are taking this journey with me. I truly love hearing from you and so value your comments and feedback that so often help and teach me, which in turn we can help and teach other Boomers.

No matter if or when we connect, to all my dear fellow Boomers reading this book,

TAKE CONTROL OF YOUR LIFE!

Don't let another year pass you by...take control of your destiny...and most definitely, don't accept what people tell you. There is a great big life for you in your next years and you deserve to live it with all the well-deserved gusto you can.

And lastly, always remember:

We are the Baby Boomers and We Will Change Aging in America.

You'll see.

—Mitzi

About the Author
Mitzi Beach

Mitzi Beach, ASID CAPS, is an award-winning professional Interior Designer and Boomer Expert. She is the owner of Mitzi Beach Interiors with expertise in sizing interiors to meet changing life stages. Mitzi also specializes in connecting big brands to the Boomers—the fastest-growing market in America. As a public speaker, blogger, and author, Mitzi inspires Boomers to live their best life now. She is happily married with nine grandchildren and resides in Wichita, Kansas, with her husband Bob and Maltese, Tess.

Mitzi Beach
www.MitziBeach.com